Physical Medicine and Rehabilitation

Neck and Back Pain

Jeffrey A. Saal, M.D.
Guest Editor

Volume 4/Number 2　June 1990
HANLEY & BELFUS, INC.　Philadelphia

STATE OF THE ART REVIEWS

Publisher: HANLEY & BELFUS, INC.
               210 South 13th Street
               Philadelphia, PA 19107

PHYSICAL MEDICINE AND REHABILITATION: State of the Art Reviews   (ISSN 0888-7357)
Volume 4, Number 2   (ISBN 1-56053-029-4)

PHYSICAL MEDICINE AND REHABILITATION: State of the Art Reviews is published triannually (three times per year) by Hanley & Belfus, Inc., 210 South 13th Street, Philadelphia, Pennsylvania 19107.

POSTMASTER: Send address changes to PHYSICAL MEDICINE AND REHABILITATION: State of the Art Reviews, Hanley & Belfus, Inc., 210 South 13th Street, Philadelphia, PA 19107.

The 1990 subscription price is $66.00 per year U.S., $76.00 outside U.S. (add $40.00 for air mail). Single copies $29.00 U.S., $32.00 outside U.S. (add $10.00 for single copy air mail).

CONTENTS

It is common knowledge among many obstetricians that a significant number of women develop low back pain during pregnancy. In spite of the high prevalence of backache during pregnancy, the literature dealing with the subject is not extensive. To this day, in many pregnant patients the pathogenesis of low back pain remains obscure and a uniform therapeutic approach is still lacking. Current knowledge about the presentation and the management of this disorder is discussed in this article.

The term "whiplash" has gained widespread acceptance among the laity and the legal community, both for its euphonic as well as descriptive qualities. However, as a medical synonym it continues to languish in favor of the more accepted but also more cumbersome *acceleration-hyperextension cervical spine injury*. In either instance the pain and subsequent disability remain the same. Expeditious and appropriate treatment continue to depend on an accurate anatomic-pathologic diagnosis and an appropriate therapeutic regimen.

Passive movement techniques are an important aspect of the total physical therapy program for patients with symptoms of cervical origin. Many concepts presented in this chapter are based upon the Australian approach, because the author's background in the manual therapies was influenced by the philosophies and training of Geoffrey Maitland. Maitland was a pioneer in the development of a methodical examination for the selection of passive movement techniques.

This chapter introduces the concept and basis of cervicothoracic stabilization training. Traditionally, the patient with cervicothoracic pain has been treated with cervical collars, cervical traction, ultrasound, electric stimulation, soft tissue massage, and joint mobilization. Although these techniques may form an integral part of the early treatment process, they also rely more heavily on the practitioner than on active patient participation.

There are very few non-life-threatening illnesses that generate as much emotion in the health care provider as does back pain in the injured worker. The first section of this article discusses the scope of the problem and reviews several cost-impact studies as demonstrable examples. Next is an epidemiologic and behavior profile of the stereotypical injured worker. The third section addresses the assessment and diagnostic evaluation of the injured worker. Lastly, the management of the worker with back pain is discusssed.

The future of spinal medicine appears bright and exciting. However, it will require the dedication of exceptional physicians and scientists to the study of painful spinal disorders. Additionally, it will require the teaming of appropriately trained physiatrists, surgeons, radiologists, psychiatrists, anesthesiologists, internists, physical therapists, and chiropractors into a multi-disciplinary effort directed towards solving this complex spectrum of problems.

CONTRIBUTORS

Joseph P. Farrell, M.S., P.T.
Owner, Redwood Orthopaedic Physical Therapy, Inc., Castro Valley, California; Senior Clinical Faculty, Kaiser Orthopedic Physical Therapy Residency Program, Hayward, California

Avital Fast, M.D.
Associate Professor of Rehabilitation Medicine, New York Medical College, Valhalla, New York; Chairman, Department of Rehabilitation Medicine, St. Vincent's Hospital and Medical Center, New York, New York

Stanley A. Herring, M.D.
Private Practice, Puget Sound Sports Physicians, Seattle, Washington; Clinical Assistant Professor, Department of Rehabilitation Medicine, and Clincal Assistant Professor, Department of Orthopaedics, University of Washington, Seattle, Washington

Richard J. Herzog, M.D.
Co-Medical Director, NeuroSkeletal Imaging Center, San Francisco Spine Institute, Daly City, California

Myron M. LaBan, M.D., F.A.C.P.
Clinical Associate Professor, Wayne State Universeity, Detroit, Michigan; Director, Department of Physical Medicine and Rehabilitation, William Beaumont Hospital, Royal Oak, Michigan

Carol P. Prentice
Alexander Technique Teacher, San Francisco, California

Jeffrey A. Saal, M.D.
Director, Research & Education, San Francisco Spine Institute, Daly City, California; Assistant Professor, University of California, Irvine, Irvine, California

Joel S. Saal, M.D.
Physiatrist, San Francisco Spine Institute, Daly City, California

John L. Shelton, Ph.D.
Adjunct Assistant Professor, University of Washington; Staff, Valley Medical Center, Seattle, Washington

Mark J. Sontag, M.D.
Physiatrist, San Francisco Spine Institute, Daly City, California

Tara Sweeney, P.T.
Physical therapist, San Francisco Spine Institute, Daly City, California

James N. Weinstein, D.O.
Associate Professor, Department of Orthopaedic Surgery; Director, Spine Diagnostic and Treatment Center, University of Iowa Hospitals and Clinics, Iowa City, Iowa

Stuart M. Weinstein, M.D.
Private Practice, Puget Sound Sports Physicians; Clinical Instructor, Department of Rehabilitation Medicine, University of Washington School of Medicine, Seattle, Washington

PUBLISHED ISSUES, 1987–1989

1990–1991 ISSUES

**Rehabilitation and
the Aging Population**
Edited by F. Patrick Maloney, M.D.
and Kevin M. Means, M.D.
Little Rock, Arkansas

The Coma Emerging Patient
Edited by Elizabeth Sandel, M.D.
and David W. Ellis, Ph.D.
Camden, New Jersey

Amputations and Prostheses
Edited by Lawrence W. Friedman, M.D.
East Meadow, New York

Musculoskeletal Pain
Constance D. Schwab, M.D.
Chicago, Illinois

Neck and Back Pain
Edited by Jeffrey A. Saal, M.D.
San Francisco, California

Rehabilitation of Chronic Pain
Edited by Nicolas E. Walsh, M.D.
San Antonio, Texas

**The Adult with Early Onset
Disability**
Edited by Daniel Halpern, M.D.
South Chatham, Massachusetts

Pediatric Rehabilitation
Gabriella Molnar, M.D.
Oakland, California

Subscriptions and single issues available from the publisher—Hanley & Belfus, Inc.,
Medical Publishers, 210 South 13th Street, Philadelphia, PA 19107 (215) 546-7293.

PREFACE

Back pain and neck pain are major areas of concern for physiatrists. This issue of PM&R: STARs presents important and practical information to help unravel the spinal pain dilemma.

I lead off the issue with a chapter on advances in nonoperative treatment of intervertebral disc herniation. The next chapter by Dr. Joel Saal on inflammation focuses on the biomechanical events that may lead to pain and to the degenerative changes that occur in the intervertebral disc. Then Dr. James Weinstein's chapter on neurophysiology of pain describes the exciting direction in which pain research is heading. However, this information must be placed in perspective alongside the psychologic and experiential aspects of pain. In all these chapters compelling evidence is assembled that nonoperative treatment is almost certainly the wave of the future.

Diagnostic imaging of the spine has made tremendous advances in recent years. The chapter by Dr. Richard Herzog contains a very complete discussion of the current state of the art in spinal imaging, with emphasis on high resolution multiplanar computed tomography and magnetic resonance imaging. This chapter should serve as a gold standard to all practitioners of spinal medicine.

The dilemma of the injured worker looms heavily over the medical care system. Low back pain is the leading cause of musculoskeletal disability in this group of patients. The chapters by Sontag and Stuart Weinstein et al. review important and provocative material relevant to this area of spinal medicine.

Dr. Avital Fast's chapter tackles the neglected area of low back pain related to pregnancy. He presents a likely mechanism by which such low back pain may occur and discusses why certain therapeutic interventions may be preferable over others.

Neck pain following vehicular trauma is the subject of Dr. Laban's chapter. His discussion of injury mechanisms and rehabilitation techniques provides many useful guidelines in the care of these patients.

Manual medicine remains a mystery for many practitioners. The chapter by Joseph Farrell is a useful review to place manipulative treatment by physical therapists into focus. However, it does not address the important issues of chiropractic manipulative treatment, which deserves further study and discussion.

Cervicothoracic stabilization represents an advance in the rehabilitation of painful neck and upper back disorders. The program outlined in the chapter by Sweeney et al. is easy to follow and implement. It was written as a practical presentation, with a brief overview of the theoretical construct on which it is based.

The final chapter is an editorial by this author that attempts to address the future direction of spinal medicine. The excellent presentations in this book act as an appropriate spring board for such a discussion. This book represents a varied group of key topics relevant to the practice of spinal medicine. We hope it will be a welcome addition to the shelf of any health care provider interested in the subject of spinal pain.

JEFFREY A. SAAL, M.D.
GUEST EDITOR

JEFFREY A. SAAL, MD

INTERVERTEBRAL DISC HERNIATION: ADVANCES IN NONOPERATIVE TREATMENT

From the San Francisco Spine
 Institute
Daly City, California

Reprint requests to:
Jeffrey A. Saal, MD
San Francisco Spine Institute
1850 Sullivan Ave., #140
Daly City, CA 94015

Lumbar intervertebral disc herniation is a common cause of low back pain and radiculopathy. Although more than 50 years have passed since Mixter and Barr's initial reports,[21] controversy still exists regarding indications for surgical intervention and the appropriate surgical procedure of choice. Disc extrusion has been considered a condition best dealt with by surgical intervention,[1,25–27] and weakness often is still considered an indication for surgery despite the favorable outcome reported by Weber.[29,30] Consequently, the role of nonoperative management of this clinical condition remains open for debate.

The presence of lateral stenosis as a reason for failed lumbar disc surgery is well described by Burton et al.[3] It is, therefore, apparent that patients having herniated discs with stenosis fall into a separate and distinct clinical subtype from patients having herniated discs without stenosis, and that each possesses different outcomes requiring different therapeutic approaches and surgical decision-making criteria. Therefore, if lateral canal stenosis is not adequately addressed by the surgical approach, the patient has a high degree of likelihood of becoming a surgical failure. Previous studies have not distinguished patients with or without stenosis accompanying their herniated intervertebral discs.[1,8,14,18,23,25–27,29–31]

In addition, there have been studies suggesting that surgically treated patients with herniated discs have had a more favorable outcome in the first year than nonsurgically treated patients.[16,29,30] This information has been used in an attempt to rationalize early surgical intervention.

We undertook a study in an attempt to determine whether patients with lumbar disc herniation and radiculopathy without stenosis could be treated effectively with aggressive conservative care. Additionally, we wished to determine the recovery time of our patients in order to clarify whether surgical patients or nonoperative patients fared better during the initial weeks and months of treatment.

Our study group consisted of patients with seemingly acceptable surgical indications as reported in previous studies. These indications included extruded discs, neurologic weakness, and failure to improve with conservative measures such as bed rest, traction, and therapeutic exercise. Disc extrusion was defined as radiographic evidence of nuclear material that had migrated beyond the confines of the outer fibers of the annulus fibrosis. If the disc material was contained by the posterior longitudinal ligament and had migrated inferior or superior to the disc space, it was considered an extrusion as well. A sequestered fragment was considered to be present when there was no sign of contiguous connection of the fragment with the disc proper. Contained herniations were defined as nuclear material still contained by the confines of the outer annulus.

Also in the study group were a group of patients who were advised by a surgeon that surgical intervention was absolutely necessary and should not be delayed. These patients had been instructed by the examining surgeon that surgery was indicated to prevent further neurologic deterioration, and furthermore the patients were told that any delay in surgical intervention could lead to an irreversible neurologic deficit. This information was given to these patients despite the lack of any literature to support this contention. Additionally, Weber's 10-year study clearly demonstrated that patients with neurologic deficit fared as well as patients without neurologic loss.[30]

Following the nonoperative treatment study, we planned a prospective study to evaluate the natural history of extruded discs that had not been surgically removed or enzymatically altered by chemonucleolysis. Prior to this study there had not been a study to adequately assess this phenomenon. There have been isolated reports documenting regression of herniated discs.[12,17] Spangforte's computer-assisted analysis of surgically treated disc herniations concluded that disc extrusions were best treated surgically. Although not documented, the concern that perithecal and perineural fibrosis will develop secondary to disc extrusions has commonly been used as an argument for prompt surgical treatment.[7] Moreover, there have been concerns regarding neurological recovery if nuclear extrusions are left to deform the neural structures over a prolonged period.[14] However, there are no specific data to support these conclusions.

The purpose of the second study was to evaluate the natural history of morphologic changes within the lumbar spine in patients who sustained lumbar disc extrusions. All patients in this study were treated nonoperatively for radicular pain and neurologic loss. The following questions were addressed: (1) Does perithecal or perineural fibrosis result when extrusions are not removed surgically? And (2) do disc extrusions spontaneously resolve and, if so, how rapidly?

MATERIALS AND METHODS

Study 1

The available records of patients seen at our spine clinic with a diagnosis of herniated lumbar intervertebral disc between January 1, 1985 and April 1,

1986 were reviewed. Patients who met the following criteria were included in the study group:

1. Those with an available computed tomography (CT) scan and/or magnetic resonance imaging (MRI) data with radiologic interpretation of "herniated nucleus pulposus."
2. Those with a diagnosis of lumbar radiculopathy based on:
   (a) A primary complaint of leg pain and a secondary complaint of back pain supported by a similar pattern on a patient-completed pain diagram.
   (b) A positive electromyogram (EMG) study demonstrating the electrophysiologic presence of lumbar radiculopathy.
   (c) A positive straight leg raising test reproducing leg pain at less than 60° elevation.
   (d) An aggressive treatment program, undergone by all patients, that included: back school; exercise training to teach spinal stabilization, i.e., dynamic maintenance of postural control, trunk and general upper and lower body—strengthening exercises; and flexibility exercises.

Epidural injections and/or selective nerve-root blocks were used when indicated for pain control. The underlying premise of the program was that the patient undergo active, not passive, treatment. Criteria that excluded patients from the study group were:

1. Previous lumbar surgery, and
2. The presence of significant stenosis or spondylolisthesis as noted on a CT scan or MRI scanning (significant stenosis, defined as a minimum of a Grade 3 on the Glenn Scale[10]).

All CT and MRI scans were reviewed by the authors for confirmation of diagnostic findings. Patients with contained herniations versus extruded fragments were noted (disc herniation, defined as a focal posterior disc abnormality of at least 5 mm). Data collected from a patient chart review included:

1. The history of the chief complaint of leg and back pain
2. The patient-completed pain diagram
3. The duration of the symptoms
4. A history of request for second opinion regarding surgery
5. The patient's work status at the time of initial evaluation
6. Physical exam findings of weakness and straight leg raising
7. EMG test results.

A standardized questionnaire including questions from the Oswestry Scale,[6] pain self-rating, work status, and self-rating of outcome was mailed to each patient who met the above criteria. Patients were additionally asked if they underwent either subsequent surgical or nonoperative treatment after completing our program. Self-rating criteria were as follows:

1. Excellent: working full-time, performing usual athletic activities.
2. Good: working full-time but limited in performance of athletic activities.
3. Fair: working part-time only, unable to participate in athletic activities.
4. Poor: unable to work and unimproved following treatment.

Out of a total of 347 consecutively identified patient records reviewed, 64 were included in the group to whom questionnaires were mailed. Exclusion criteria included the diagnostic factors mentioned above and nonavailability of patient CT scans. All questionnaires not returned within 3 weeks from the initial mailing resulted in a repeated mailing with a letter requesting completion. If no response was obtained by the second mailing, follow-up phone calls were made and the questionnaire was completed. A total of 58 questionnaires were returned—a 91% response rate.

Data analysis included calculation of:

1. Rates of return to work
2. Average sick-leave time
3. Subsequent surgery due to failure of conservative care
4. A self-rating outcome.

Rates were calculated for the entire study population; a comparison between the workers' compensation patients and private pay patients was made; and contained versus extruded herniations were noted. Separate rates of outcome were determined for the group of patients seeking a second opinion regarding surgery.

Study 2

The study population consisted of a patient group previously evaluated in our nonoperative treatment trial. All of these patients had documented disc extrusions and radiculopathy. All had a primary complaint of leg pain, and all had a positive straight leg raising reproducing their leg pain at less than or equal to 60 degrees. Additionally, 87% had muscle weakness on a neurologic basis in a root level distribution corresponding to the site of disc disease. All patients with disc extrusion from the previous study were contacted, and nine agreed to participate in the study and to undergo a follow-up imaging examination. An additional two patients who satisfied the study criteria but were not subjects of the nonoperative study were also included.

Computed tomographic examinations were obtained on all patients at the inception of treatment. These studies were compared to follow-up MRI studies. The initial CT scans were evaluated for the following criteria: disc size and position, thecal sac effacement, nerve root enlargement or displacement, and evidence of central or intervertebral canal stenosis. In addition to the pathomorphology evaluated on the CT scans, follow-up MRI studies also evaluated disc hydration at the herniated and contiguous levels, and the presence of perithecal or perineural fibrosis. The following grading system was utilized to evaluate change in fragment size on the follow-up studies:

Grade 1. 0 to 50% decrease in size
Grade 2. 50 to 75% decrease in size
Grade 3. 75 to 100% decrease in size.

RESULTS

Study 1—Nonoperative Patients

Of a total of 52 nonoperative patients, 50 (those with "Good" or "Excellent" outcomes) were considered successes (85 ± 5.2% of the entire study population; 96% of all nonoperative cases). Forty-eight patients returned to work (83 ± 5.2% of the entire study population; 92 ± 3.5% of all nonoperative patients; 44 (85 ± 5%) of all of the patients returned to their previous jobs. The average sick-leave time required by patients in this group was 3.8 ± 1.0 months. Twenty-six patients (50 ± 6.9%) reported less than 1 week sick-leave (Table 1).

TABLE 1.   Summary of Data

	Percent return to work (%)	Sick leave (mos)
Total study population (n = 58)	93	4.6 ± 1.1
Nonoperative treatment subgroups		
Subgroup having extruded discs (n = 13)	100	2.9 ± 1.4
Surgical second opinion subgroup (n = 15)	100	3.4 ± 1.7
Workers' compensation subgroup (n = 11)	86	9 ± 3.3

Study 2

The results on follow-up of MRI examinations are as follows:

I. Residual fragment size:

Grade	No. of Discs	Percent
Grade 1	2	11%
Grade 2	4	36%
Grade 3	5	46%

II. Associated Morphologic Changes

	No. of Discs	Percent
Fibrosis (perithecal or perineural)	0	0%
Progression of stenosis	1	9%
Disc desiccation		
1. Level of disc herniation	11	100%
2. Contiguous levels	0*	0%
Decrease in neural impingement	11	100%

* All discs normally hydrated

The interval between the initial presentation and follow-up was a median of 25 months with a range of 8 to 77 months.

The maximum of shrinkage of the extrusions occurred in the cephalocaudal dimension. This was always associated with a reduction in neural element displacement and swelling (Fig. 1). Lesser degrees of shrinkage were noted in the AP dimension of the disc material. The largest extrusions decreased the most in size and had the greatest likelihood of total resolution (Fig. 2).

The two cases that decreased the least were the smallest extrusions and had the shortest interval between initial presentation and follow-up scan, 16 and 8 months, respectively. Notably, both of these patients reported clinical improvement with no significant leg pain or disability at time of follow-up.

DISCUSSION

These studies demonstrate that patients with herniated nucleus pulposus and radiculopathy can be successfully treated nonoperatively. Their sick-leave time and return-to-work rates were superior to those reported in previous studies for patients suffering the same complaints who were treated surgically. The data from our two studies do not support the contention that surgery is a more efficacious method for treating patients with herniated nucleus pulposus.

However, there may be individual circumstances where surgery offers advantages over nonsurgical management. The timeline for expected improvement during a regimen of nonsurgical treatment must be monitored closely. At the start of treatment, patients should be instructed that herniated nucleus pulposus

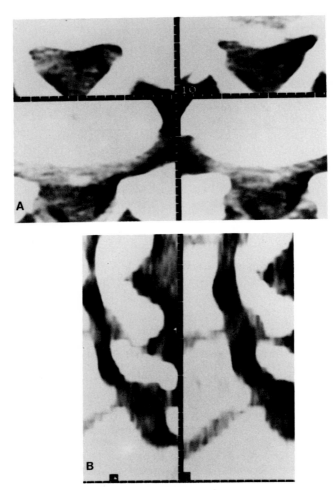

FIGURE 1. On the axial *(A)* and sagittal *(B)* images from a multiplanar CT study, there is a large sequestered disc fragment positioned caudal to the L5–S1 disc level in the right lateral recess. *(Figure continued.)*

has an excellent prognosis and that they can expect an equal chance of success within similar timelines whether they choose nonsurgical or surgical care at the initiation of treatment. During the first month of treatment, an improvement of 30–50% in patient function and a comparable reduction in pain are to be expected. By the end of the second month of treatment, an improvement of 70–80% should have been achieved. If a patient's progress does not meet these timelines, clinical improvement through the nonsurgical program can be expected to be very protracted or not successful. Therefore, at 8 weeks, all cases should be carefully assessed. Patients who are not progressing according to the goals outlined should be given the option to proceed with surgery. They should be told that surgery will probably achieve the expected successful result more rapidly than continuing the nonoperative program, considering the lack of progress in the first two months

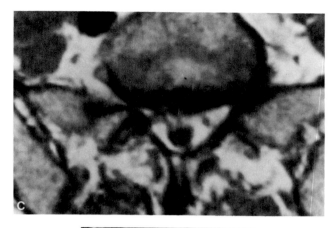

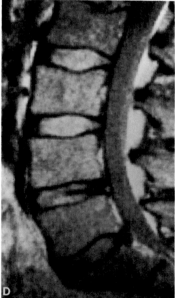

FIGURE 1 *(continued)*. On the followup MR study on the T1-weighted axial *(C)* and the proton density-weighted sagittal *(D)* images at the L5–S1 disc level, there is only a small posterior midline disc protrusion and no evidence of a sequesetered disc fragment.

of nonoperative care. Patients should also be instructed that nonsurgical care is still appropriate, but that a decision to continue their nonsurgical care program must be reconsidered in the light of their desires and time constraints.

When trying to decide on the surgical candidacy of a patient, the following information should be considered. The presence of weakness did not adversely affect outcome in the group with herniated nucleus pulposus in our study. Disc extrusion was successfully managed in 13 out of 15 cases (87%). Improvement occurred well within the first year as noted by the average sick-leave time. Four

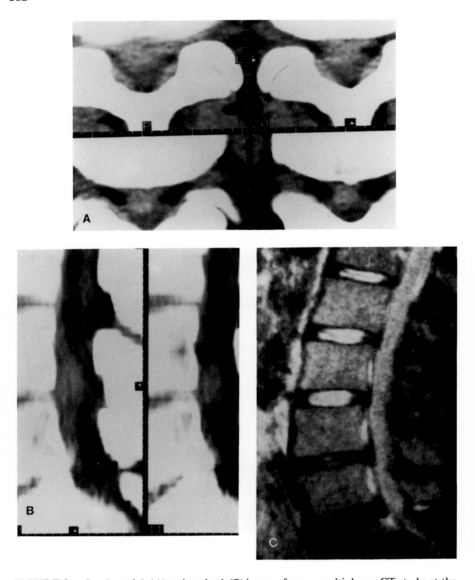

FIGURE 2.   On the axial *(A)* and sagittal *(B)* images from a multiplanar CT study at the L4–5 disc level there is a large extruded disc fragment. In the followup MR study on a T2-weighted sagittal image *(C)*, there is only a small posterior disc protrusion at the L4–5 disc level along with disc degeneration. At the L5–S1 disc level, a new disc extrusion is identified.

out of six patients who failed nonoperative treatment were found to have stenosis at subsequent lumbar spine surgery. It appears that herniated nucleus pulposus combined with stenosis carries a different prognosis than herniated nucleus pulposus alone. Our study on the natural history of extruded discs demonstrated that extruded lumbar intervertebral discs have the capacity to resolve without surgical extirpation or chemonucleolysis and identified a need for further study of the precise mechanism of resorption.

Theoretically, resorption begins when the nuclear material is exposed to the vascular supply of the epidural space and is separated from the nutrient supply of the disc. The separation of the extruded fragment from the disc may preclude the production and replenishment of the hydrophilic proteoglycan in the disc, thereby leading to progressive desiccation. Additionally, cellular elements in the epidural space stimulated by the inflammatory response may promote phagocytes of the offending nuclear material. Inflammation and neovascularization of the extrusion may maintain the hydration level initially. However, as the inflammation subsides, neovascularization may lead to phagocytes and resorption.[13,19]

On MR studies, extruded or sequestered disc fragments may demonstrate increased signal intensity when compared to the disc from which they originated.[20] This phenomenon may be secondary to ingrowth of granulation tissue or alternatively may be due to water inhibition by the extruded nuclear material. Theoretically, as a result of herniation an abrupt decrease in compressive and tensile forces acting on the disc could result in a change in the equilibrium between the swelling pressure of the herniated fragment and the external forces.[28] This could result in increased water inhibition by the extruded disc, resulting in increased disc fragment size. The increased hydration of the extrusion could account for the increased signal intensity frequently identified on the T2-weighted MR images when the signal intensity in the extrusion is compared to the disc of origin.[22]

The pain associated with nuclear extrusions may result from the inflammatory component rather than from compression.[9,28] This phenomenon can be explained by the recent demonstration of high levels of phospholipase A_2, a potent pro-inflammatory enzyme, in human lumbar disc herniations.[24] It is unclear whether resorption of the extrusion coincides with clinical improvement. Corticosteroid introduced into the epidural space will inhibit the liberation of inflammatory mediators and the inflammatory response, thereby controlling pain generation. It may, theoretically, speed the resorption process.[10,15]

Total resorption of the largest extrusions was most often observed in our disc extrusion study. The distance by which the extruded fragment is separated from the corresponding facet may play an important role in the loss of nutrition and subsequent phagocytosis and resorption. It is important to note that no follow-up scans of the fragments demonstrated fibrosis resulting from the disc extrusion. In these cases, conservative nonsurgical management of disc extrusions did not lead to the delayed sequela of perithecal or perineural fibrosis. Prompt resolution of inflammation plays a key role in limiting the extent of fibrotic reaction.[11] It is therefore evident that only surgical trauma is capable of causing extensive fibrosis in the epidural space. Postoperative healing occurs in the presence of the ingrowth of granulation tissue, which is itself an inflammatory reaction destined to resolve by a fibrotic reaction.

We have clearly demonstrated the efficacy of nonoperative care of lumbar disc herniation. We have also shown that the natural history of extruded nuclear material causing radiculopathy is favorable. Among the questions that remain are the central issues of which therapeutic exercise regimen and which aspects of nonsurgical care are most effective in the treatment of this condition and why. The exercise program used in our study involves strengthening certain muscle groups to enhance dynamic stabilization of the spine. The following five questions address aspects of exercise regimens that need to be evaluated when these programs are used in the treatment of patients with lumbar disc herniation.

Would aerobic exercise itself be sufficient?[5]

It is our contention that unless the lumbar intervertebral disc is protected from repetitive microtrauma in the acute stage, continued nuclear migration with a concomitant inflammatory reaction will occur, thereby prolonging the clinical syndrome of radicular pain. If mechanical stresses that increase intradiscal pressure are allowed to continue, the natural process of nuclear resorption will be delayed. This delay may led to neural complications such as intraneural venous congestion, leading to intraneural edema and axonal anoxia.

We therefore attempt to ensure the protection of the functional spinal segment via dynamic lumbar muscular stabilization training. If patients are merely instructed to train aerobically, they may develop improved cardiorespiratory fitness but will not be able to protect their intervertebral discs from repetitive injury. Pain suppression may be a dividend of aerobic conditioning via excitation of the endorphin analgesic mediated system, but underlying lumbar disease will remain untreated. Aerobic exercise can only be offered to the aerobically deconditioned patients whose leg pain is not severe enough to limit their participation. If one considers that the chief complaint of a patient with a herniated nucleus pulposus is radicular leg pain that limits activity, the prescription of aerobic exercise in the acute stage of treatment appears irrational. If one initially prescribes bed rest to quell acute radicular symptoms, this will result in loss of muscle strength, soft tissue contractures, and loss of total body calcium. If one then asks one's patients to begin an aerobic training program, this would subject them to significant risk of injury. Moreover, a common problem encountered is patients who continue to reinjure themselves due to improper preaerobic stretching routines. Exercises (e.g., the hurdler's stretch and forward-bending toe touches) that force the lumbar spine into extreme degrees of flexion are often taught to patients with disastrous consequences. The flexion required by these exercises places high levels of stress on the posterior annulus fibrosis, which may lead to fatigue failure of the collagen-supporting matrix, resulting in gradual disc prolapse and nuclear herniation. There are spine-safe ways to obtain increased flexibility during flexion without compromising the intervertebral discs. These spine-safe techniques should be taught during dynamic lumbar muscular stabilization (DLMS) training.

Would a general conditioning program be as efficacious as DLMS?

Highly conditioned athletes suffer from lumbar disc injuries at a rate that does not appear to be any different than the general population. Their conditioning level alone is not sufficient to protect the lumbar intervertebral disc from injury. To simply place someone in a fitness program and not teach him or her how to stabilize the spine against mechanical stresses capable of injuring the intervertebral disc is to encourage failure. Moreover, selective strengthening of isolated muscle groups and stretching of shortened soft tissue are mandatory before the patient with a lumbar spine condition begins a fitness program. Most "conditioning" programs call for compound movements that require the large muscle groups and may ignore certain muscles (e.g., the lower oblique abdominal muscles), a situation we consistently encounter when injured athletes present with disc herniation. They may be strong, but they will be found to have isolated deficiencies in the strength of the lower abdominal musculature or spinal extensors. Poor flexibility in the hamstring musculature, hip flexors, and the hip rotator musculature is also quite common. Improving overall fitness is extremely important but must be undertaken in the context of protecting the lumbar spine. This means exercising in spine-safe postures and learning to reduce intradiscal loads while performing activities of daily living (ADLs).

Can manipulative treatment or traction "reduce" nuclear herniations, ameliorate pain, and prevent recurrences of this clinical condition?

Traction and manipulation are commonly used treatment modalities for painful spinal disorders. However, traction has not demonstrated that it can actually cause nuclear or annular relocation. Manipulative treatment can yield pain relief but is considered contraindicated in cases of neurologic loss due to herniated nuclear material. Manual treatment can be valuable for improving mobility in hypomobile spinal segments and for passively stretching contracted soft tissues. However, neither of these modalities is capable of doing anything other than offering short-term relief of pain. They do not improve the lumbar spine's ability to withstand potentially injurious loads, nor do they address the underlying disorder.

Most importantly, these modalities do not transfer the responsibility of care to the patient where ultimately it must reside. Patients cannot function as passive receptacles of care, but instead they must be active participants in their rehabilitation program. Traction and manipulation may have a place in the pain-control phase of treatment but cannot be considered effective long-term solutions to intervertebral disc disorders.

Can back education alone be successful treatment without the application of an exercise program?

Although this has not been studied, it seems reasonable to assume that simply educating patients about proper body mechanics and supplying them with adequate information for performing the techniques to acquire strength and flexibility are not satisfactory. One study that did evaluate back education in a group of first-time back pain sufferers did not demonstrate the efficacy of this approach.[2] However, the question of how much exercise training is necessary to accomplish the required result does need additional study.

What is the role of epidural corticosteroid injections?

The role that epidural corticosteroid injections plays in the treatment of herniated nucleus pulposus is open to debate. In our experience, epidural corticosteroid injections can reduce radicular referral pain associated with disc herniation more rapidly than any other treatment modality, thereby dramatically shortening the pain-control phase of treatment and allowing a prompt initiation of exercise training. We have found the caudal approach to be as effective as the translumbar for herniations at the L5–S1 interspace. However, sequestered nuclear fragments causing S1 nerve root displacement often require the addition of an S1 transforaminal nerve block. If the sequestered fragment is laterally placed, causing L5 nerve root displacement and symptoms, then it is necessary to unilaterally place a translumbar epidural injection at L5. In the case of a foraminal herniation in the exit zone or extra-foraminal zone, a transforaminal selective nerve root block (SNRB) is often necessary. Herniations at the L4–L5 interspace can be dealt with similarly. However, in cases of large central or paracentral herniations, a translumbar approach may be more effective than caudal entry. Herniations at the upper lumbar levels require a translumbar injection at the level in question.

A second epidural or SNRB can be performed as early as 1 week later if the first epidural is only partially effective. A total of three to four injections may also be necessary to achieve success in refractory cases when radicular symptoms persist and limit participation in the stabilization training program. However, the clinician must be quite certain that the injection procedures are indeed improving the functional status of the patient, thereby facilitating the patient's participation in the stabilization training program. If the procedures are only offering the patient short-term relief from pain and not facilitating progressive functional improvement, this treatment approach should be abandoned and the patient should be considered a strong candidate for surgery.

A positive prognostic sign is the disappearance of radicular pain associated with straight leg raising provoked immediately after the injection. A poor prognostic sign is the lack of improvement in crossed straight leg raising following a block procedure. In addition, a list that is not correctable after a block procedure portends a poor prognosis for recovery through nonoperative care. However, you must be certain that the epidural injection clearly instills the medication into the epidural space. This can only be guaranteed if the block procedures are administered under fluoroscopic control.

Decisions regarding injection procedures must be based upon a careful correlation of the history, physical examination, electrodiagnostic studies, and imaging results. In general, injection procedures should not be done without prior imaging tests (MRI or CT) and electrodiagnostic evaluation. We have never experienced a case of progression of neurologic deficit after an epidural injection. Some authors have hypothesized that volume expansion associated with epidural instillation of medication might cause compression of the neural elements, thereby causing an additional insult resulting in advancement of a neurologic deficit.[4] We have seen a short-term increase in patient's radicular pain after an epidural injection in the presence of large extrusions, but we have not noted any true neurologic progression. If the neurologic loss associated with a spinal lesion is due to neurapraxia, an early improvement in neurologic function is often noted following an epidural corticosteroid injection, probably related to reduction of neural element edema, thereby improving axonal transport.

Prognostic indicators must be monitored during the nonoperative treatment program. The response to epidural injection presents some strong indicators of nonoperative treatment success. In our experience, the presence of stenosis coupled with herniated nucleus pulposus does not necessarily present an indication for surgery, but instead lowers the odds for nonoperative treatment success from the 90% range to the 65% to 75% range—but this requires further study. In addition, the type, degree, and location of stenosis and its effect upon treatment are the subject of a study currently in progress at our institution.

The nonoperative treatment program we used in our study is presented in the appendix.

APPENDIX

DYNAMIC LUMBAR MUSCULAR STABILIZATION PROGRAM DESCRIPTION

Treatment Phases

1. Pain control
   a. Back first aid
   b. Trial extension exercises
   c. Trial of traction
   d. Basic stabilization exercise training
   e. NSAIDs
   f. Non-narcotic analgesics
   g. Corticosteroids
      (1) Oral
      (2) Epidural injection
      (3) Selective nerve root injection
      (4) Facet injection
2. Exercise training
   a. Soft-tissue flexibility
      (1) Hamstring musculotendinous unit
      (2) Quadriceps musculotendinous unit
      (3) Iliopsoas musculotendinous unit
      (4) Gastrocsoleus musculotendinous unit
      (5) External and internal hip rotators
   b. Joint mobility
      (1) Lumbar spine segmental mobility
      (2) Hip range of motion
      (3) Thoracic segmental mobility
   c. Stabilization program
      (1) Finding neutral position (standing, sitting)
      (2) Prone gluteal squeezes
      (3) Supine pelvic bracing
      (4) Bridging progression
         (a) Basic position
         (b) One leg raised
         (c) Stepping
         (d) Balance on gym ball
      (5) Quadruped
         (a) With alternating arm and leg movements (ankle and wrist weights are used during the progression)
      (6) Kneeling stabilization
         (a) Double knee
         (b) Single knee
         (c) Lunges (hand held weights added during the progression)
      (7) Wall slide quadriceps strengthening
      (8) Position transition with postural control
   d. Abdominal program
      (1) Curl-ups
      (2) Dead bugs

      (3) Diagonal curl-ups
      (4) Diagonal curl-ups on incline board
      (5) Straight leg lowering
  e. Gym program
      (1) Latissimus pull-downs
      (2) Angled leg press
      (3) Lunges
      (4) Hyperextension bench
      (5) General upper body weight exercises
      (6) Pulley exercises to stress postural control
  f. Aeorobic program
      (1) Progressive walking
      (2) Swimming
      (3) Stationary bicycling
      (4) Cross-country ski machine
      (5) Running
         (a) Initially supervised on a treadmill

Program Description

Pain control. Decisions for use of pain-control methods will depend on patient level of function and ability to comply with the prescribed exercise program. All patients are to be enlisted in a therapeutic exercise regimen as tolerated by their level of pain and neurologic loss. The initial stage, back first aid, involves the application of ice, resting in a position of comfort, and basic instruction in body mechanics to facilitate pain-free movement. The use of medications will be kept to a minimum. Transcutaneous nerve stimulation may also be used for pain control. Acupuncture may occasionally be used during this phase. A trial of traction (gravity inversion, pelvic traction, or auto-traction) is to be used for patients with refractory radicular pain following extension exercises. Traction will be continued in those patients who have a marked reduction of radicular pain.

    Non-narcotic analgesics (i.e., acetaminophen) and NSAIDs (nonsteroidal anti-inflammatory drugs) may be prescribed. Occasionally, a limited course (up to 2 weeks) of a class-3 narcotic analgesic such as Tylenol with Codeine may be prescribed. No patients will receive a schedule II medication, a sedative hypnotic, or a muscle-relaxant medication.

    Prescribed bed rest will not be recommended. Patients will be instructed to pursue a level of activity that does not exacerbate their radicular pain or worsen a neurologic deficit. Persistent radicular pain will be treated with corticosteroid therapy. Epidural injections will be the treatment of choice, although in some patients a tapering course of oral corticosteroids will be used. Patients with persistent back pain consistent with facet syndrome will be asked to undergo facet-joint corticosteroid injections. Injection therapy will be used to facilitate the patient's functional progress. Decisions to inject or re-inject are to be based upon the patient's ability to progress with the active exercise program.

    Exercise Training. The key element in the phase devoted to exercise training is the accomplishment of adequate dynamic control of lumbar spine forces in order to eliminate repetitive injury to the intervertebral discs, facet joints, and related structures. This training program is called "Stabilization Training." Stabilization exercise routines are to be divided into basic and advanced levels.

Prior to strengthening exercises, the focus of all exercise is soft tissue flexibility and joint range of motion. Flexibility training focuses on the musculotendinous units of the hamstrings, quadriceps, iliopsoas rectus femoris, external and internal hip rotators, and gastrocsoleus. Strict attention is to be paid to maintenance of neutral spine posture while the stretching exercises are performed. These exercises are to be carried out on a daily basis. Stretching is first performed passively by the exercise training and then is included as part of the patient's home program. Continued active assistive stretching is occasionally necessary to fully overcome soft tissue contracture that results from limited mobility and nerve root irritation.

The patient is to be trained in active joint mobilization methods, such as extension exercises in prone and standing positions, as well as alternating mid-range flexion and extension while in a four-point stance. Abdominal muscle strengthening will begin with simple "curl-ups." From this, the patient is to progress to dynamic abdominal bracing, an exercise that uses alternate arm and leg movements while lying supine, contracting the abdominal musculature, and holding the spine in neutral position. More advanced exercises will include diagonal curl-ups and diagonal curl-ups performed on an inclined board. Once the patient is able to carry out 3 sets of 15 repetitions, more challenging exercises are to be undertaken. At the end of this stage of the program, lower abdominal muscle strengthening is to be emphasized using straight leg lowering exercises.

Demonstration of proper form and technique is required for the patient to graduate from the basic level. These same guidelines are then to be applied to the weight-training portion of the program. Aerobic and anaerobic training is to be incorporated into the total fitness program. Aerobic conditioning will be initiated early in the program in the form of walking. Shortly thereafter, the patient is to be asked to ride a stationary bicycle and/or to use a cross-country ski machine. Swimming will be encouraged for those patients interested in it but is not to be uniformly used with all patients. These activities are to be first performed under supervision to ensure maintenance of neutral spine posture. Training levels are to be tailored to the patient's age, medical history, and level of aerobic conditioning according to previously established American College of Sports Medicine guidelines.

Decisions for advancement to more challenging exercises during the program will be based upon functional progress rather than pain level. The program end-point will be determined by maximal functional improvement that will not advance further by exercise training or pain control.

REFERENCES

1. Barr J, Kubik C, Molloy M, et al: Evaluation of end results in treatment of ruptured lumbar intervertebral discs with protrusion of nucleus pulposus. Surg Gynecol Obstet 125:250–256, 1967.
2. Berwick DM, Budman S, Feldstein M: No clinical effect of back schools in an HMO: A randomized prospective trial. Spine 14:338–344, 1989.
3. Burton C, Kirkaldy-Willis W, Young-Hing K, et al: Causes of failure of surgery on the lumbar spine. Clin Orthop 157:191–199, 1967.
4. Cuckler JM, Bernini PA, Wiesel W, et al: The use of epidural steroids in the treatment of lumbar radicular pain. A prospective, randomized, double-blind study. J Bone Joint Surg 67:63–66, 1985.
5. Davies JE, Gibson T, Tester L: The value of exercises in the treatment of low back pain. Rheumatol Rehab 18:243, 1979.
6. Fairbank J, Davies J, Couper J, O'Brien J: The Oswestry Low Back Pain Disability Questionnaire. Physiotherapy 66:271–272, 1980.

7. Finneson B: Low Back Pain. Philadelphia, J.B. Lippincott, 1973.
8. Frymoyer J, Hanley E, Howe J, et al: Disc excision and spine fusion in the management of lumbar disc disease. Spine 3:1–6, 1978.
9. Gertzbein S: Degenerative disc disease of the lumbar spine. Clin Orthop 129:68–71, 1977.
10. Glenn W, Rothman S, Rhodes M: Computed tomography/multiplanar reformatted (CT/MPR) examinations of the lumbar spine. In Computed Tomography of the Lumbar Spine. San Francisco, University of California Printing Department, 1982.
11. Goetzl E: Immunologic regulation of fibrosis. Rheumatol Clin Immunol (An Advanced Course). 1986, pp 151–158.
12. Guinto F Jr: CT demonstration of disk regression after conservative therapy. AJNR 5:632–633, 1984.
13. Hakelius A: Prognosis in sciatica: A clinical follow-up of surgical and nonsurgical treatment. Acta Orthop Scand 129(Suppl):5–76, 1970.
14. Hakelius A, Hindmarsh J: The comprehensive reliability of preoperative diagnostic methods in lumbar disc surgery. Acta Orthop Scand 43:234–238, 1972.
15. Hirata F, Schiffman E, Venkatasubramanian K, et al: A phopholipase A2 inhibitory protein in rabbit neutrophils induced by glucocorticoids. Proc Natl Acad Sci USA 77:2533–2536, 1980.
16. Hurme M, Alaranta H: Factors predicting the result of surgery for lumbar intervertebral disc herniation. Spine 12:933–938, 1987.
17. Kahanovitz N, Viola K, Watkins R, et al: A multicenter comparative analysis of workers' compensation and private patients undergoing surgical diskectomy. ISSLS, 1988.
18. Kambin P, Gellman H: Percutaneous lateral discectomy of the lumbar spine. Clin Orthop 174:127–132, 1983.
19. Lindblom K, Hultqvist G: Absorption of protruded disc tissue. J Bone Joint Surg 32A:557–560, 1950.
20. Masaryk T, Ross J, Modic M, et al: High-resolution MR imaging of sequestered lumbar intervertebral disks. AJNR 8:351–358, 1988.
21. Mixter W, Barr J: Rupture of the intervertebral disc with involvement of the spinal canal. N Engl J Med 211:210, 1934.
22. Modic M, Masaryk T, Ross J: Magnetic Resonance Imaging of the Spine. Chicago, Year Book, 1989.
23. Nachlas W: Research Committee of the American Orthopaedic Association: End-result study of the treatment of herniated nucleus pulposus. J Bone Joint Surg 34A:981–988, 1952.
24. Saal J, Franson R, Dobrow R, et al: High levels of inflammatory phospholipase A2 activity in lumbar disc herniation. Spine (in press).
25. Salenius P, Laurent : Results of operative treatment of lumbar disc herniation. Acta Orthop Scand 48:630–634, 1977.
26. Shannon N, Paul E: L4/5 and L5/S1 disc protrusions: Analysis of 323 cases operated over 12 years. J Neurol Neurosurg Psychiatry 42:804–809, 1979.
27. Spangfort E: The lumbar disc herniation: A computer-aided analysis of 2,504 operations. Acta Orthop Scand 142(suppl):5–95, 1972.
28. Urban J, McMullin J: Swelling pressure of the lumbar intervertebral discs: Influence of age, spinal level, composition, and degeneration. Spine 13:179–187, 1988.
29. Weber H: Lumbar disc herniation: A prospective study of prognostic factors including a controlled trial, Part I. J Oslo City Hosp 28:33–61, 1978.
30. Weber H: Lumbar disc herniation: A controlled prospective study with ten years of observation. Spine 8:131–140, 1983.
31. Wilson D, Harbaugh R: Microsurgical and standard removal of the protruded lumbar disc: A comparative study. Neurosurgery 8:422–424, 1981.

JOEL S. SAAL, MD

THE ROLE OF INFLAMMATION IN LUMBAR PAIN

From the San Francisco Spine
   Institute
Daly City, California

Reprint requests to:
Joel S. Saal, MD
San Francisco Spine Institute
1850 Sullivan Avenue, #140
Daly City, CA 94015

Although back pain and disc degeneration are common in the population at large, the factors underlying (or initiating) disc degeneration and the mechanisms of pain generation remain undefined.[4,48] It has been generally assumed that mechanical factors alone are responsible for the generation of pain. However, the concept of the "clinically significant disc lesion" as one that physically impinges upon pain-sensitive neural structures is too insensitive to explain the majority of disc lesions encountered in daily clinical practice. The use of sophisticated imaging techniques reinforces this concept. Frequently, patients with radicular pain or radiculopathy will have no neural impingement noted on MRI scan. Although physical forces clearly play a role in disc-mediated nerve root injury and radicular pain, it is equally clear that a role exists for chemically mediated injury. The clinical features of a given individual patient can be analyzed in terms of their chemical or mechanical components. Individual patients may manifest more chemical or mechanical symptoms depending upon the natural history of their disc lesion. The physical and biochemical components of disc disease develop in parallel, not individually. These changes as well as the clinical features of an individual patient follow the degenerative cascade as described by Kirkaldy-Willis.[31]

PATHOPHYSIOLOGY OF LUMBAR DISC DEGENERATION

The existing body of knowledge indicates that degeneration of the lumbar disc, either directly or indirectly, is central to the clinical construct of lumbar spine pain. Separation of the cartilagenous endplate and loss of distinction between the borders of the annulus fibrosis within the annulus fibrosis of the disc are the earliest observable pathoanatomic changes of disc degeneration.[31,56,67] Progression of the fissures with loss of supporting strength of the annulus follows. This eventually results in herniation of nuclear disc.[31]

There is experimental evidence to indicate that the "herniated" material may represent metaplastic annular tissue that is part of an attempted repair process.[38,39] Tears of the annulus, and diffuse or focal protrusion of the annulus are other morphologic abnormalities of the disc observed in both symptomatic and asymptomatic individuals.[27,70] Contiguous tissues that exhibit degenerative changes that parallel disc changes include zygoapophyseal joint arthrosis and ligamentum flavum thickening, both of which cause nerve canal stenosis.[31,67] Although the bony changes usually parallel the changes in disc morphology, the bony adaptation to stress may occur in the absence of observable disc abnormality. The chemical alterations that evolve in the degenerating disc are in part responsible for the altered morphology of the disc and contiguous tissues as degeneration progresses.

There are two basic cell populations within the intervertebral disc. The predominant cell type within the outer annulus fibrosis is a fibrocyte type, similar to those found in mature tendon or ligament. The nucleus pulposus is sparsely cellular, with chondrocyte-like cells as the predominant cell type.[25] These cell populations are responsible for maintenance of the matrix of the nucleus and annulus, as well as the structural integrity of the annular collagen envelope.[70] The limited blood supply to the inner annulus and nucleus creates a unique situation for the disc in terms of maintenance of its internal milieu, with the cells exhibiting limited turnover.[65] As in articular cartilage, some of the chondrocytes have a life span as long as adult life. In skeletally mature discs, the cells of the inner annulus appear to have the highest level of metabolic activity,[1,2,38,56] approximating one-fifth of an articular cartilage chondrocyte.[40]

The process of disc degeneration and herniation have been associated with alterations of the biochemical balance and cellular activity of the disc.[1,2,62] In degenerative disc, chondrocyte clones similar to those observed in osteoarthritic articular cartilage are noted.[67] As in osteoarthritic cartilage, these may represent an attempted repair process. The matrix concentration of proteoglycan and the degree of proteoglycan aggregation decrease as a disc degenerates.[38,46,50] The normal collagen/proteoglycan interaction, considered to be protective of both substances, is disturbed or altered in degenerating discs.[1,38,46] This may expose attack sites for the degrading enzymes present in the matrix.[2,62] In degenerating discs, the ratio of collagen type I to collagen type II in the nucleus and the annulus changes, as does the amount of elastin, especially in the border region between annulus and nucleus.[24,29] These changes are capable of degrading the extracellular matrix. Activation of and change in substrate type for collagenase (change from type II to type I collagen) and elastase have been observed in degenerative and herniated lumbar discs.[52] This process has been studied in animal simulations as well as human surgical and autopsy specimens. Additionally, the pH of degenerative painful discs has been noted to be more acidic than those of normal discs.[47,48]

It is not known whether or not these biochemical changes and enzymic alterations are a consequence or precipitating factor in disc degeneration or herniation. The events that trigger these changes in the chemical constituents of the disc are not known. However, it is clear that there is a system of enzymatic activity that is carefully balanced to maintain the normal homeostasis of the intervertebral disc. The morphologic changes of disc degeneration are accompanied by changes in this enzymatic balance. The reaction of cells to their environment, both physical and biochemical, is in part reflected by these altered enzymatic relationships. It is attractive to consider that an altered balance in enzymatic activity can produce degradation products capable of initiating an inflammatory response in neighboring nerve tissue. An analogous situation exists in osteoarthritis of a typical diarthrodial synovial joint. The proteoglycan fraction released from the cartilage as a result of degeneration induced by changes in the action of synovial fluid enzymes causes an inflammatory reaction in synovium. The substances directly responsible for the putative chemically induced nerve injury may be the enzymatic breakdown products or the enzymes themselves.[6] There are other components of the biochemical balance of the intervertebral disc that play a role in this phenomenon.

Our studies of phospholipase A2 (PLA2) activity in surgical samples of human herniated discs demonstrated extraordinarily high levels in comparison to other models of inflammation.[61] This neutral pH active, calcium-dependent phospholipase not only regulates the arachidonic acid cascade, but is also inflammatory in its own right.[13,68] Indeed, both steroidal and nonsteroidal anti-inflammatory medications are directed at control of the arachidonic acid cascade and/or PLA2 expression.[14] PLA2 has been demonstrated to play a role in numerous models of inflammation, including inflammatory synovial effusion.[57,66] Inflammatory intermediates (eicosanoids) have been demonstrated to be capable of direct nociceptive stimulation.[35,55] As powerful mediators of inflammation, the eicosanoid compounds (prostaglandins, leukotrienes, and 15 lipoxygenase products) have that capability. The Ca 2+ dependent, neutral pH active PLA2 plays a role as a regulatory enzyme, carefully controlled by cellular factors.[13] Interleukin-1 (IL-1) has been demonstrated to stimulate PLA2 production by articular cartilage chondrocytes.[19]

Numerous investigators have implied an association between immunological phenomena and aspects of inflammation in lumbar disc disease.[5,16,17,20,41,42,49,51,53,60] Naylor and co-workers suggested a humoral immune response secondary to disc prolapse, and possibly responsible for disc degeneration.[51] Altered cell mediated immunity was strongly suggested by the experimental findings of Bobechko and Hirsch,[5] and further supported by the demonstration of altered leukocyte migration and transformation by Gertzbein and others.[10,16,17] However, none of these investigators was able to demonstrate a specific antibody reaction. Marshall, et al.[41] coined the term *chemical radiculitis* to imply nerve injury on the basis of chemical factors associated with lumbar disc injury. Marshall suggested a systemic humoral antibody response to disc injury based upon the experimental findings of serum antibodies to human disc material from patients with a recent history of back pain. The consensus of thought was that there was an autoimmune response to disc extrusions and exposed nuclear material, but a clear demonstration of inflammation and of the components of the pathway involved was lacking.

Histopathological findings compatible with inflammation of a variable degree in nerve root specimens and disc samples obtained at surgery have also been documented.[20,25,26,36] The demonstration of persistently altered fibrinolytic activity in patients with chronic back pain suggests a role for chronic inflammation, but no direct link to inflammation as an etiology was shown.[32] The capacity for nucleus pulposus in both human and animal lumbar discs to act as an antigen has been shown, with the proteoglycan fraction suggested as a probable source.[54] That the proteoglycan fraction may have the capacity to act as an antigen may explain the experimental findings of variable degrees of cellular infiltrate in response to transplanted autologous nucleus in the epidural space of rabbits.[42] These findings suggested a role for inflammation in degenerated and unclassified disc abnormalities with unexplained pain. The combined weight of this experimental evidence is suggestive of a biochemical source for nerve injury in lumbar disc disease. The presence of inflammation in this situation and the specific biochemical mechanism are demonstrated by the finding of elevated levels of PLA2 activity in surgical cases of human lumbar discogenic radiculopathy.

The beneficial therapeutic effect of epidural injection of corticosteroids, as well as local anesthetic alone, can be explained by PLA2 inhibition by anesthetics and the inhibitory action of corticosteroids on PLA2. There is a class of pharmacologic agents of various chemical families currently in development that consists of inhibitors of PLA2 activity. Moreover, the rapid, positive effect of chymopapain may be explained in part by proteolytic action on the PLA2 molecule.

Investigations of the inflammatory nature of intervertebral disc material have been inconclusive. Exposure of rabbit tibial nerve to disc material resulted in no greater conduction abnormality than mechanical deformation alone,[59] but autologous disc material injected into the epidural space of canines[42] caused histologic evidence of an inflammatory response.

The focus of the literature described above has been upon the role of an immune response in the production of symptoms and as a cause of degeneration of lumbar intervertebral discs. It is important to distinguish between an immune response and the process of inflammation. This is especially important when considering the experimental evidence presented in the literature, as the evidence demonstrates a role for inflammation but not necessarily for an immune response. An immune response consists of a programmed set of chemical and cellular events triggered by a foreign substance capable of acting as an antigen.[22,30] An autoimmune response occurs when a part of the human body acts as the antigen. The immune response involves the presentation of the antigen by a macrophage to T lymphocytes, with the subsequent triggering of antibody production by B lymphocytes and interaction of the complement cascade, with resultant cytotoxic reactions and leukocyte infiltration.[30] The latter part of this process results in inflammation. However, inflammation can occur in the absence of this full-blown immune response.[12,15,30,37] Injury or foreign substance may cause the elaboration of chemical mediators (monokines and cytokines) on the part of macrophages and monocytes, with the subsequent generation of inflammatory mediators.[7,8,11,21,30,37]

The demonstration of inflammation in human lumbar disc disease, be it injury, herniation, or disc degeneration, has important clinical implications. These certainly include considerations regarding treatment of this condition, as well as our understanding of the mechanisms involved in the pathogenesis of the clinical findings. The frequently encountered paradox of the structural abnormalities being inadequate (partially, if not wholly) to explain the clinical findings is clarified by the aforementioned biochemical events.

HYPOTHESIS ON THE PATHOPHYSIOLOGY OF LUMBAR RADICULOPATHY CAUSED BY HERNIATED NUCLEUS PULPOSUS

We speculate that the initial result is at the interface of the intervertebral disc and the epidural space occurring as the result of a loss of integrity of the outer annulus. This injury results in the triggering of a local inflammatory response. The initiation of inflammation may be due to the escape of high local concentrations of inflammogenic material into the epidural space on a gross (extruded fragment) or microscopic level (leakage from a degenerating disc). Phospholipase A2 within the nucleus pulposus could serve as the inflammogenic material by increasing the local production of eicosanoids and other inflammatory mediators. Stimulation of a cellular reaction by nuclear material to release PLA2 into the epidural space may also occur.

Local production of inflammatory mediators can cause nerve inflammation and swelling as well as altered electrophysiologic function.[33,68] The liberation of prostaglandins and leukotrienes has been demonstrated to cause sensitization of small neurons, and it also enhances pain generation.[34,35,45,55] Further membrane injury could directly result from the direct action of PLA2 on susceptible tissue.[13,68] Altered vascular permeability in response to inflammatory mediators may result in venous congestion and intraneural edema.[13,64] A normal conduction by nerve fibers and generation of pain not necessarily caused by nerve compression follow. Intraneural ischemia and enhanced axonotmesis may also occur.[13,64] The further insult of mechanical deformation of neural elements by central or intervertebral canal stenosis may magnify the degree of nerve injury. Intraneural ischemia and more widespread wallerian degeneration of axons would result. We have observed a higher degree of injury in the combined presence of both lumbar intervertebral disc herniation and stenosis.[60] Further study is necessary to confirm the validity of this hypothesis.

The clinical implications of these findings are similar to our growing insight into the etiology and treatment of cardiovascular disease. In each instance, the resulting structural abnormalities are clear. We seek to understand the biochemical processes giving rise to the observed pathoanatomy. If the basic abnormality in radiculopathy caused by lumbar disc herniation is as much a problem of biochemical perturbation as it is one of pathological anatomy, attention focused primarily on surgical solution rather than on chemical intervention appears shortsighted.

A purely mechanical construct inadequately explains the cause of disc degeneration, as well as many clinical cases of discogenic pain syndromes and radiculopathy. The mechanism of lumbar radiculopathy is commonly considered to be due to impingement of disc tissue on the neural structures.[58] However, in many surgically treated lesions, no physical pressure on the spinal nerve by disc material is observed at the time of surgery.[44] Imaging by computed tomography or magnetic resonance may fail to demonstrate adequate structural abnormality of the disc to explain symptoms that appear too discogenic. Signs of lumbar radiculopathy with corresponding abnormal EMG examinations are not infrequently observed in patients with minimal morphologic abnormalities.

This is further supported by experiments in which ligatures placed around noninflamed nerve roots created paresthesia only, but pressure placed on inflamed nerve roots caused pain in the same experimental subjects.[44,63] As a corollary to this, in many cases of disc herniation or protrusion, there is no clear relationship between the extent of the morphologic abnormality and the degree of symptoms or nerve injury. Following the intradiscal administration of chymopapain, clinical improvement is noted long before any morphologic change is observed. In some of these situations, no significant morphologic change occurs at all.[23,43] Similarly, with percutaneous nuclectomy, no observable morphologic change of the disc is noted to accompany significant improvement in the clinical findings and symptoms. Epidural local anesthetic injection alone or in combination with corticosteroid may have a dramatic temporary (and occasionally permanent) benefit in situations of radiculopathy from disc herniation in the absence of any subsequent pathoanatomic changes.[9]

Clearly, something other than a morphologic abnormality of the external disc architecture is the source of the nerve injury and symptom production in discogenic pain subsets, and in cases of discogenic radiculopathy. These observations may be explained by peptide changes in the dorsal root ganglion,[69] or ephaptic transmission in this structure.[28] Alternatively, there may be mechanical factors present within the intradural connections of the nerve root that are not visible by means of external imaging.[3]

However, a proinflammatory chemical source within the disc capable of stimulating annular nociceptors and causing inflammation of the spinal nerve can explain all of these observations. The findings of extraordinarily high levels of PLA2 in painful degenerative discs may explain the mechanism of nerve root injury and pain generation, as well as constitute a component of the biochemical pathway of disc degeneration. This enzyme can be normally produced by chondrocytes,[19] and this may occur in the active regions of the disc, possibly under the regulation of IL-1.[18,19] As an initiating or associated event in disc degeneration, the loss of control of endogenous suppressors of PLA2 may cause elevated levels of PLA2 activity.[13] In human synovial fluid, the enzyme activity was associated with an endogenous protein inhibitor of the PLA2.[68] The relationship of PLA2 to its endogenous suppressor may be further disrupted by the changes of pH that occur in the process of disc degeneration.[13,48] Loss of control of this regulatory enzyme results in an increased activity that results in expression of PLA2's inflammatory capability, by production of proinflammatory mediators as well as the direct inflammatory action of PLA2. PLA2 can cause membrane injury directly, and by production of free radicals capable of lipid peroxidation resulting in increased membrane phospholipid breakdown.[13] This activity has not been tested on peripheral nerve membrane. This could explain pain production from discs with no significant morphologic abnormality. The role of substance P in pain generation linked to inflammation may occur as a result of the neuropeptide's effect on prostaglandin production.[69]

Attempts at a pharmacological interruption of the degenerative inflammatory process are needed. Further investigation of regulatory parameters of the response is also indicated. The interface of immunology and biochemistry in lumbar disc disease has arrived. New evidence suggests that attempts at control of a chemical process by a chemical solution seem more logical than a purely structural approach.

REFERENCES

1. Bayliss M, Johnstone B, O'Brien J: Proteoglycan synthesis in the human intervertebral disc variation with age, region, and pathology. Spine 13:972–981, 1988.
2. Bayliss MT, Urban JPG, Johnstone B, et al: In vitro method for measuring synthesis rates in the intervertebral disc. J Orthop Res 4:10–13, 1986.
3. Beel JA, Stodiek LS, Luttges MW: Structural properties of spinal nerve roots: Biomechanics. Exp Neurol 91:30–40, 1986.
4. Biering-Sorenson F: Low back trouble in a general population of 30- 40- 50- and 60-year-old men and women: Study design representatives and basic results. Dan Med Bull 29:288–299, 1982.
5. Bobechko WP, Hirsch C: Autoimmune response to nucleus pulposus in the rabbit. J Bone Joint Surg 47B:574–580, 1965.
6. Brandt K: Osteoarthritis. Rheumatology and Clinical Immunology: An Advanced Course, 1988.
7. Chang J, Gilman SC, Lewis AJ: Interleukin 1 activates phospholipase A2 in rabbit chondrocytes: A possible signal for IL1 action. J Immunol 136:1283–1287, 1986.
8. Chrisman OD, Ladenbeauer-Bellis LM, Fulkerson JP: The osteoarthritic cascade and associated drug actions: Osteoarthritis Symposium. Sem Arth Rheumatol 11:145, 1981.
9. Cuckler JM, Bernini PA, Weissel SW, et al: The use of epidural steroids in the treatment of lumbar radicular pain: A prospective, randomized, double-blind study. J Bone Joint Surg 67A:63–66, 1985.
10. Elves MW, Bucknill T, Sullivan MF: In vitro inhibition of leukocyte migration in patients with intervertebral disc lesions. Clin Orthop North Am 6:59–65, 1975.
11. Evans CH: Cellular mechanism of hydrolytic enzyme release in osteoarthritis. Sem Arth Rheumatol 11:93–94, 1981.
12. Famaey J: Phospholipases, eicosanoid production and inflammation. Clin Rheumatol 1:84–94, 1982.
13. Franson R, Raghupathi R, Fry M, et al: Inhibition of human phospholipases A2 by cis-unsaturated fatty acids and oligomers of prostaglandin B1. In Mukherjee (ed): Biochemistry, Molecular Biology, and Physiology of Phospholipases A2 and Their Regulatory Factors. New York, Plenum (in press).
14. Franson RC: Isolation and characterization of a phospholipase A2 and inflammatory exudate. J Lipid Res 19:18–23, 1978.
15. Franson RC, Patriarca P, Elsbach P: Phospholipid metabolism by phagocytic cell: Acid and alkaline phospholipases associated with rabbit polymorphonuclear leukocyte granules. J Lipid Res 15:380–388, 1974.
16. Gertzbein SD: Degenerative disc disease of the lumbar spine: Immunological implications. Clin Orthop Rel Res 129:68–71, 1977.
17. Gertzbein SD, Tile M, Gross A, Falk R: Autoimmunity in degenerative disc disease of the lumbar spine. Orthop Clin North Am 6:67–73, 1975.
18. Gilman SC, Berner PR, Chang J: Phospholipase A2 activation by interleukin-1: Release and metabolism of arachidonic acid by IL-1 stimulated rabbit chondrocytes. Agents Action 21:345–347, 1987.
19. Gilman SC, Berner PR, Mochenm E, et al: Interleukin-1 activates phospholipase A2 in human synovial cells. Arthritis Rheum 31:126–130, 1986.
20. Goldie I: Granulation tissue in the ruptures intervertebral disc. Acta Orthop Scand 22:302–304, 1959.
21. Greaves MW, Camp RD: Prostaglandins, leukotrienes, phospholipase, platelet activating factor, and cytokines: An integrated approach to inflammation of human skin. Arch Dermatol Res 280(Suppl):33–41, 1988.
22. Harris EAJ: Scientific Rationale for Future Treatment of Rheumatoid Arthritis. Rheumatology and Clinical Immunology: An Advanced Course, 1988.
23. Heithoff K: Computed tomographic assessment of the postoperative spine. Spine Update 243–269, 1984.
24. Herbert CM, Lindberg KA, Jayson MIV, Bailey AJ: Changes in the collagen of human intervertebral discs during aging and degenerative disc disease. J Mol Med 1:79–91, 1975.
25. Hirsch C: Studies on the pathology of low back pain. J Bone Joint Surg 41B: 237–243, 1959.
26. Hirsch C, Shajowicz F: Studies on structural changes in the lumbar annulus fibrosis. Acta Orthop Scand 22:184–231, 1952.
27. Hitselberger WE, Witten RM: Abnormal myelograms in asymptomatic patients. J Neurol 28:204–206, 1968.
28. Howe JF, Loesser JD, Calvin WH: Mechanosensitivity of dorsal root ganglia in chronically injured axons: A physiologic basis for the radicular pain of nerve root compression. Pain 3:25–41, 1977.

29. Johnson EF, Chetty K, Moore LM, et al: The distribution and arrangement of elastic fibres in the intervertebral disc of the adult human. J Anat 135:301–309, 1982.
30. Kelley WN, Harris ED, Ruddy S, Sledge CB: Textbook of Rheumatology. Philadelphia, W.B. Saunders, 1985.
31. Kirkaldy-Willis WH, Wedge JH, Yong-Hing K, Reilly L: Pathology and pathogenesis of lumbar spondylosis and stenosis. Spine 3:319–328, 1978.
32. Klimiuk PS, Pountain GD, Keegan AL, Jayson MIV: Serial measurements of fibrinolytic activity in acute low back pain and sciatica. Spine 12:925–928, 1987.
33. Lampert PW: Mechanism of demyelination in experimental allergic neuritis. Lab Invest 20:127–138, 1969.
34. Levine JD, Lau W, Kiniat G, et al: Leukotriene B4 produces hyperalgesia that is dependent on polymorphonuclear leukocytes. Science 225:743–745, 1984.
35. Levine JD, Taiwo Y, et al: Hyperalgesic properties of 15 lipoxygenase products of arachidonic acid. Proc Natl Acad Sci 83:5331–5334, 1986.
36. Lindahl O, Rexed B: Histologic changes in spinal nerve roots of operated cases of sciatica. Acta Orthop Scand 20:215–225, 1951.
37. Lindblad S, Hedfors E: Arthroscopic and immunohistologic characterization of knee joint synovitis in osteoarthritis. Arthritis Rheum 30:1081–1088, 1987.
38. Lipson J, Miur H: Proteoglycans in experimental intervertebral disc degeneration. Spine 6:194–210, 1981.
39. Lipson SJ: Metaplastic proliferative fibrocartilage as an alternative concept to a herniated intervertebral disc. Spine 13:1055–1060, 1988.
40. Maroudas A, Stockwell RA, Nachemson A, Urban J: Factors involved in the nutrition of the human lumbar and intervertebral disc: Cellularity and diffusion of the glucose in vitro. J Anat 120:113–130, 1975.
41. Marshall LL, Trethewie ER, Curtain CC: Chemical radiculitis: A clinical, physiological and immunological study. Clin Orthop Rel Res 129:61–67, 1987.
42. McCarron RF, Winjed MW, Hudgins PG, Laros GS: The inflammatory effect of nucleus pulposus: A possible element in the pathogenesis of low back pain. Spine 12:760–764, 1987.
43. McCulloch JA: An approach to the patient with sciatica. Spine Update 19–22, 1984.
44. McNab I: The mechanism of spondylogenic pain. Pain 89–95, 1971.
45. Mense S: Sensitization of Group IV muscle receptors to bradykinin by 5-hydroxytryptamine and prostaglandin-E2. Brain Res 225:95–105, 1981.
46. Mitchell PEG, Handry NGC, Billewicz WZ: The chemical background of intervertebral disc prolapse. J Bone Joint Surg 43B:141–151, 1961.
47. Nachemson AL: Intradiscal measurements of pH in patients. Acta Orthop Scand 40:23–42, 1969.
48. Nachemson AL: The lumbar spine: An orthopaedic challenge. Spine 1:59–71, 1976.
49. Naylor A: The biochemical aspects of disc degeneration and prolapse. In Intervertebral Disc Herniation and Degeneration. England, Proceedings of the Royal Academy of Surgery, 1962.
50. Naylor A: Intervertebral disc prolapse and degeneration: The biomechanical and biophysical approach. Spine 1:108–114, 1976.
51. Naylor A, et al: Enzymic and immunologic activity in the intervertebral disc. Orthop Clin North Am 6:51–58, 1975.
52. Ng SC, Weiss TB, Quennel R, Jayson MIV: Abnormal connective tissue degrading enzyme patterns in prolapsed intervertebral discs. Spine 11:695–701, 1986.
53. O'Brien JA, Jaffray D: Isolated intervertebral disc resorption: A source of mechanical and inflammatory back pain? Spine 11:397–401, 1986.
54. Pankovitch AM, Korngold L: A comparison of the antigen properties of nucleus pulposus and cartilage protein polysaccharide complexes. J Immunol 99:431–437, 1967.
55. Pateromichelakis S, Rood JP: Prostaglandin E2 increases mechanically evolved potentials in the peripheral nerve. Experientia 37:282–284, 1981.
56. Pritzker KP: Aging and degeneration in the lumbar intervertebral disc. Orthop Clin North Am 8:66–77, 1977.
57. Pruzanski W, Vadas P, Stefanski E, Urowitz MB: Phospholipase A2 activity in sera and synovial fluids in rheumatoid arthritis and osteoarthritis. Its possible role as a proinflammatory enzyme. J Rheumatol 12:211–216, 1985.
58. Rydevik B, Brown MD: Pathoanatomy and pathophysiology of nerve root compression. Spine 9:7–15, 1984.
59. Rydevik B, Brown MD, Ehira T, et al: Effects of graded compression and nucleus pulposus on nerve tissue: An experimental study. Acta Orthop Scand 54:670–671, 1983.

60. Saal JA, Saal JS: The nonoperative treatment of herniated nucleus pulposus with radiculopathy: An outcome study. Spine 14:431–437, 1989.
61. Saal JS, Franson RC, Dobrow R, et al: High levels of inflammatory phospholipase A2 activity in lumbar disc herniations. Spine (in press).
62. Sedawofia KA, Tomlinson IW, Weiss JB, et al: Collagenolytic enzyme systems in human intervertebral disc: Their control, mechanism, and their possible role in the initiation of biomechanic failure. Spine 7:213–222, 1982.
63. Smyth MJ, Wright V: Sciatica and the intervertebral disc: An experimental study. J Bone Joint Surg 40A:1401–1418, 1958.
64. Sunderland S: Nerves and Nerve Injuries. New York, Churchill Livingstone, 1978.
65. Urban J, Holm S, Maroudas A, Nachemson A: Nutrition of the intervertebral disc: Effect of fluid flow on solute transport. Clin Orthop 170:296–302, 1982.
66. Vadas P, Pruzanski W, Kim J, Fornasier V: The proinflammatory effect of intra-articular injection of soluble human and venom phospholipase A2. Am J Pathol 134:807–811, 1989.
67. Vernon-Roberts B: The pathology and interrelation of intervertebral disc lesions, osteoarthritis of the apophyseal joints, lumbar spondylosis, and low back pain. In The Lumbar Spine and Back Pain. London, Pitman Publishing, 1980.
68. Vishwanath B, Fawzy A, Franson R: Edema inducing activity of phospholipase A2 purified from human synovial fluid and inhibition by aristolochic acid. Inflammation 12:549–561, 1988.
69. Weinstein J, Claverie W, Gibson S: The pain of discography. Spine 13:1344–1348, 1988.
70. Wiesel SW, Tsourmas N, Feffer HL, et al: A study of computer assisted tomography. I. The incidence of positive CAT scans in an asymptomatic group of patients. Spine 9:549–551, 1984.

JAMES N. WEINSTEIN, D.O.

RECENT ADVANCES IN THE NEUROPHYSIOLOGY OF PAIN

From the Spine Diagnostic
 and Treatment Center
Department of Orthopaedic
 Surgery
University of Iowa Hospitals
 and Clinics
Iowa City, Iowa

Reprint requests to:
James N. Weinstein, DO
Director, Spine Diagnostic
 and Treatment Center
Department of Orthopaedic
 Surgery
University of Iowa Hospitals
 and Clinics
Iowa City, Iowa 52242

Seventeenth century French philosopher René Descartes wrote of the existence of the specific pathways for transmitting pain information from an injured part of the body through the spinal cord to a pain center in the brain. This "telephone-cable" view of how pain messages are transmitted has been accepted for many years. The fact that transection of this "cable" will not consistently alleviate the pain reveals a very important message about the generation of pain itself. Pain is a complex perception and depends not only on the intensity of stimulus but on the situation one has experienced, and more importantly upon the component parts of the individual who is experiencing the stimulus. Thus, it may be and often is a very subjective experience. In one culture young men are asked to cross rivers with grappling hooks embedded in their stomachs to prove their manhood. In viewing pictures of these men, it is certainly not obvious that they are in pain. However, the expression of pain and the severity of pain differ from one individual to another.

Since the days of Descartes, a great deal of information has been accumulated in order to gain further understanding of how messages from injured tissue reach the brain. However, little information about the location in the brain where final decisions are made as to whether something is painful or not is available. In addition, little is known regarding the cortical mechanisms involved in one's perceptions of back pain.

DEFINITION

Before discussing the neuroanatomy of the functional spinal unit, it is important to have a definition of pain. The Taxonomy Committee of the International Association for the Study of Pain (1979) defined pain as "an unpleasant sensory and an emotional experience associated with actual or potential tissue damage, or described in terms of such damage."[1] The Committee went on to say that pain is always subjective. Each individual learns, over time, the application of the word pain through experiences related to injury in early life. Pain often occurs in the absence of tissue damage and may in some instances be an emotional experience. If one regards his or her experience as painful and reports it in the same way as pain caused by direct tissue damage, then it should be accepted as painful. Thus, pain does not always have to be linked directly to a damaging stimulus.

The limitations of the verbalization of low back pain are, as we know, restricted. Unfortunately, back pain is what the patient feels and how he or she expresses those feelings to us.

The very nature of back pain and its impact upon industrialized countries have imposed a sense of urgency for a better understanding of pain pathways and neural mechanisms. Treatment modalities and related approaches are so varied across health care workers that appropriate analysis of efficacy has at best been difficult. Today, if one method of treatment fails, another method is tried and, if it fails, a further method is tried; it is therefore hard to study the natural history of any one condition or the result of any one specific treatment.

NEUROANATOMY OF THE FUNCTIONAL SPINAL UNIT

Dorsal primary rami provide nerve fibers that innervate each functional spinal unit of the lumbar spine. The distribution of medial branches from each dorsal ramus of the spinal nerve sends fibers to the vertebral periosteum, facet joints capsules, and ligamentous connections of the neural arches. The sinu-vertebral nerve provides innervation to structures within the spinal canal. Most authors agree[2-5] that the dorsal primary ramus is a branch off the spinal nerve just distal to the dorsal root ganglion and/or the dorsal section of the gray autonomic communicating ramus. Bogduk[6] and Parke[7] used dissections to show that each sinu-vertebral nerve supplies at least two intervertebral discs. The inferiorly directed branch ramifies over the dorsum of the disc at the level of entry, whereas the longer superior branches course along the lateral margin of the posterior longitudinal ligament to reach the disc of the next superior level (Fig. 1).

The posterior longitudinal ligament is the most highly innervated structure in the functional spinal unit, with both complex encapsulated nerve endings and numerous poorly myelinated free nerve endings. Undoubtedly, the elevation of this highly innervated thin strap of connective tissue may be a significant component in the production and perception of low back pain associated with lumbar disc herniations.

The sinu-vertebral nerve pain fibers have been demonstrated by both clinical and laboratory experimentation. Direct stimulation of the posterior longitudinal ligament is known to elicit back pain in humans. Pederson[8] showed that stimulation of these tissues in cats resulted in changes in blood pressure and respiration similar to those elicited by painful stimuli in other areas of the body.

The nerve endings associated with the sinu-vertebral nerve and the posterior primary ramus of each functional spinal unit have been studied by various

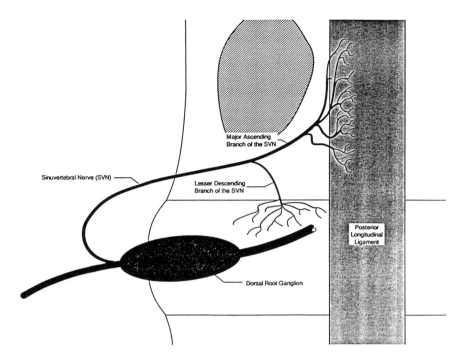

FIGURE 1. Schematic: Demonstrating the sinu-vertebral nerve, which provides innervation to structures within the vertebral canal. The sinu-vertebral has an ascending branch innervating the posterior longitudinal ligament and a lesser descending branch that also sends fibers to the posterior longitudinal ligament and annulus of the disc.

investigators.[9–11] Three types of myelinated nerve endings have been identified: (1) free nerve endings terminating as single tapered tips, (2) complex unencapsulated endings usually terminating in multiple branches with expanded tips, and (3) encapsulated nerve endings of the Vater-Pacini type. Unmyelinated perivascular nerve networks have also been described. Malinsky identified two types of perivascular nerve endings in the immature annulus fibrosis: (1) simple, free terminations of thin nerve fibers along capillary walls; and (2) more complex branchings of thicker nerve fibers within blood vessel walls.[10] In addition, plexiform and free unmyelinated nerve fiber terminals, not associated with blood vessels, are present. The structure of these various nerve endings significantly influences the type of sensation perceived, as well as its intensity.[4] Plexiform and freely ending unmyelinated nerve fibers respond to chemical or mechanical abnormalities and form the pain or "nociceptive" receptor system.

Encapsulated endings appear to be located primarily in the facet joint capsules and in the soft tissues along the anterolateral surfaces of the annulus fibrosis.[9,11] The joint capsules also have free nerve endings and complex encapsulated endings. The anterior and posterior longitudinal ligaments, the supraspinous ligaments, and the interspinous ligaments have free nerve endings and complex unencapsulated endings.[9,12] The posterior longitudinal ligament

TABLE 1. Distribution of Peripheral Nerves to the Three-Joint Complex and Surrounding Soft Tissues

Fiber Type	Function	Location
Myelinated		
Free	Tissue or joint position	Facet joint capsules; anterior and lateral surfaces of annulus fibrosus; anterior/posterior longitudinal ligaments; supraspinous/intraspinous ligaments; periosteum
Complex unencapsulated	Tissue or joint position	Same as listed above
Complex encapsulated	Pressure	Facet joint capsules; anterior and lateral surfaces of annulus fibrosus; periosteum
Unmyelinated		
Perivascular	Vasomotor	Cartilage endplates; vertebrae; blood vessels
Simple	Vasosensory	
Complex	Nociceptor	
Free	Chemical Mechanical	Annulus fibrosus; facet joint capsules; ligaments
Plexiform	Nociceptor	

appears to have the greatest number of nerve endings.[13] The cartilage endplates have perivascular nerves only.[12] The vertebral periosteum is well supplied with free endings and complex unencapsulated nerve endings,[14] and the vertebra has perivascular nerves as well as occasional solitary nerves (Table 1).[15] As stated previously, a number of investigators have reported that the peripheral layers of the annulus fibrosis have free fiber endings, but they did not find nerves in the inner regions of the annulus fibrosis or nucleus pulposus.[9,10,12,16] However, Shinohara reported free nerve fiber endings in the inner regions of the annulus and nucleus pulposus of degenerated discs.[17] Other authors[13] indicate that although unmyelinated nerves are present in fetal and neonatal disc, these nerves rapidly disappear with aging and growth. Thus, no nerves are present in the substances of normal mature human intervertebral disc material. Ultrastructural investigations, likewise, have failed to identify nerves in the inner annulus of the normal disc.

In the peripheral nervous system, three types of nerve fibers are found that transmit information from the body to the spinal cord and up to the brain.[18] The largest peripheral nerves, called A-beta fibers, are from 5–12 μm in diameter. These respond to nonnoxious, noninjurious, and nonpainful stimuli. Because of their diameter, they transmit information very rapidly to the spinal cord from the peripheral tissues. A second type of fiber is called A-delta fibers. They range from 1–5 μm in diameter and transmit information much slower due to their smaller diameter. The smallest fibers, however, are the unmyelinated C—fibers. They are less than 1 μm in diameter and transmit information even slower than the A-delta fibers. The A-delta and the C-fibers are predominantly nociceptors; i.e., they respond to injurious mechanical and/or thermal stimuli, as well as endogenous neurogenic and nonneurogenically released chemicals from damaged tissue. When you bump your elbow, the first sharp pain you experience is due to the A-delta fibers, whereas the second, diffuse, throbbing, possibly burning pain is transmitted by the C-fibers. One must remember that small C-fibers are exclusively activated by painful stimuli. However, large-diameter fibers must be

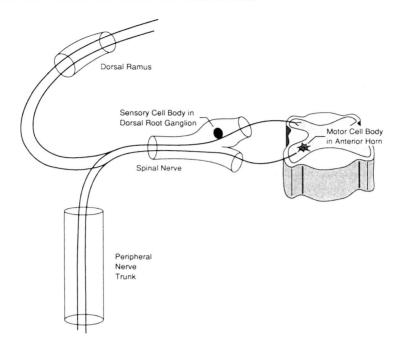

FIGURE 2.   Schematic: *Nerve roots* arising from anterior horn cells and dorsal horn nerve roots from sensory cell bodies in the dorsal root ganglion form the spinal nerve. Beyond the dorsal root ganglion, the dorsal primary ramus and peripheral nerve trunk continue.

present and play a significant role in appreciation of the quality of the stimuli to be preserved. In the absence of large fibers such as A-delta, a damaging stimulus might only be perceived as a burning sensation.

THE DORSAL ROOT GANGLION

As we move toward the spinal cord (central nervous system), from peripheral nerves to the spinal nerve, we encounter the dorsal root ganglion, the 'brain' of the functional spinal unit[19] (Fig. 2). Lindbloom and Rexed[20] were the first to implicate the dorsal root ganglion as the modulator of low back pain. Their cadaveric studies focused on compression of the dorsal root ganglion as a result of dorsolateral lumbar disc protrusions. In some specimens, enlarged facet joints were found to be an accessory factor in causing nerve injury. Such bony enlargement no doubt can cause similar damage to the dorsal root ganglion quite independent of a disc herniation. Today the importance of this compression is still uncertain.

The cells of the dorsal root ganglion were originally divided into two classes according to their diameters.[21] The large cells give rise to the large myelinated A-beta fibers, whereas the small cells give rise to the unmyelinated C-fibers and finely myelinated A-delta fibers. The central terminations of these primary afferent fibers, derived from the small ganglion cells, are primarily, but certainly not exclusively, in the substantia gelatinosa or lamina II of the dorsal horn of the spinal cord.

The dorsal root ganglion is the producer of several neurogenic peptides, including calcitonin gene-related peptide and substance P. Calcitonin gene-related peptide is the most abundant peptide discovered, to date, in the dorsal root ganglion.[22] A great deal of information is available on the blood supply to the spinal cord, but little has been written about the blood supply to the dorsal root ganglion.[23] Its vascular supply, both venous and arteriole, must play a significant role in its function. Bergman and Alexander suggested that aging and concomitant vascular changes of the dorsal root ganglion are associated with degeneration and changes in vibratory sensation. Because of the ganglion's vascular supply and tight capsule, Rydevik and associates[24] have suggested that mechanical compression of the ganglion may result in intraneural edema and a subsequent decrease in cell body blood supply, accounting for abnormal dorsal root ganglion activity and pain. In the spinal stenosis model of Delamarter, neurogenic claudication appeared to begin with venous congestion of the nerve roots and dorsal root ganglion, distal to the constricting band.[25]

Anatomically, the dorsal root ganglion serves as a vital link between the internal and external environment and the spinal cord. The primary sensory role of the spinal cord is to receive afferent stimuli in the form of action potentials and to relay the information transmitted to and from the brain. This particular mechanism of pain transmission has attracted much attention. The classic hypothesis that the effects of nerves on target organs (bone, muscle, ligaments, cartilage) are mediated by chemicals released from those nerves was first studied in the peripheral nervous system and has now proven to be valid in the central nervous system as well.[26,27] Thus, the dorsal root ganglion remains a vital link between the intrathecal spinal nerve and the extrathecal peripheral nerve.[26,27] Nervi nervorum located on the dorsal root ganglion, as well as peripheral nerves, are mechanically sensitive nociceptors themselves. Therefore, the epineurium of the doral root ganglion may be directly activated by compression or mechanical stimulation of these nociceptors. These epineurally located nociceptors appear to respond in a similar way to cutaneous nociceptors in the peripheral nervous system.[27]

Recently, a study to assess the role of the dorsal ganglion in modulating the pain response associated with discography was reported.[28] Lumbar discography is a commonly employed diagnostic tool, but important questions about it remain unresolved. Why is an abnormal discogram painful in one patient and not in another? This study was performed to investigate the changes in substance P (SP) and vasoactive-intestinal peptide (VIP), found in the dorsal root ganglion, following discography in normal and abnormal canine lumbar intervertebral discs. The data from this study suggest that dorsal root ganglion SP and VIP are indirectly affected by manipulations of the intervertebral disc. It may be that various neurochemical changes within the intervertebral disc are expressed by sensitized (injured) annular nociceptors, and in part modulated by the dorsal root ganglion. Therefore, the concomitant pain sometimes associated with an abnormal discogram image may in part be related to the chemical environment within the intervertebral disc and the sensitized state of its annular nociceptors. In this study immunohistochemical identification of SP, VIP and calcitonin-gene related peptide was made, for the first time, in the outer annulus.

ANATOMY OF THE LUMBAR NERVE ROOTS

Nerve roots constitute the anatomic and physiologic connection between the central and peripheral nervous system. Anatomically, the nerve roots pass through confined spaces in the spine where pathological changes can cause mechanical deformation. Unlike peripheral nerves, nerve roots are structurally different in both their anatomy and vascularity.[29,30] Therefore, nerve roots do not react to compression in the same fashion as peripheral nerves. Nerve roots are far less homogenous structures than are peripheral nerves. A nerve root in the lumbar spine is not a single structure or entity but rather a complex arrangement consisting of the motor root, the sensory root, and at exit through the neural foramen, the dorsal root ganglion. The nerve roots in the spinal cord are enclosed by a thin, rich sheath. Outside the sheath is cerebral spinal fluid and the spinal meninges. For each nerve root, the subarachnoid space ends at or about the level of the dorsal root ganglion. It is at the dorsal root ganglion junction that the sensory nerve fibers mix with the motor fibers to form the spinal nerve. The dura is transformed at this point to be the epineurium of the peripheral nerve. The basement membranes that originate from the root sheath itself and the layer beneath the spinal dura and arachnoid form the perineurium of the spinal nerve, which continues to become a peripheral nerve. It should be noted that nerve roots within the cauda equina lack perineurium and only have a very sparse epineurium (Fig. 3). They, therefore, may be more susceptible to compressive forces than peripheral nerves. On the other hand, nerve roots are surrounded by cerebral spinal fluid and meninges that have significant mechanical properties.[31] The dorsal sensory roots are larger in diameter than the ventral motor roots. These roots vary in length from 6 cm to 17 cm, increasing from the L1 to S1 level.[32] The axons making up the dorsal and ventral roots are extensions of the dorsal sensory root ganglion and ventral horn motor cells of the spinal cord, respectively. The survival of these axons depends on the integrity of their parent cell bodies and the various axonal transport mechanisms.

NERVE MECHANICS AND FUNCTION

Peripheral nerves respond to local compression by a total neural component reaction. At low pressure levels of 30–50 mmHg, the first effect seen in a peripheral nerve is stagnation of venous blood flow.[33] In the rabbit tibial nerve, this was seen in the 20–30 mmHg pressure range. Prolonged compression at such levels induces retrograde effects on the nutritive blood flow in the capillary circulation of nerve fascicles. As the amount of pressure and the duration of pressure increase, axonal transport becomes affected and finally complete ischemia of the nerve is seen.[33] Depending upon the duration of compression, blood flow may be restored; however, postcompression edema within the endoneurium may have a negative effect on nerve function by either altering inoic balance or by increasing the pressure within the nerve fascicles.[29]

Rydevik and his colleagues have speculated that long-standing edema can result in interneuronal fibrotic scar tissue where mast cells and fibroblasts may play a role.[34] The neurophysiological events related to nerve root compression indicate that nerve roots might be more susceptible to compression than peripheral nerves.[35,36] Rydevik's group has also pointed out that the endoneurial vessels of nerve roots and, in particular, the dorsal root ganglia are more permeable to plasma proteins than are the endoneurial vessels of peripheral nerves. There is then no effective blood-nerve barrier in nerve roots. In the peripheral nervous system the perineurium can act as a diffusion barrier to macromolecules, whereas nerve roots lack this layer and are therefore relatively more exposed to substances and agents circulating within the blood and

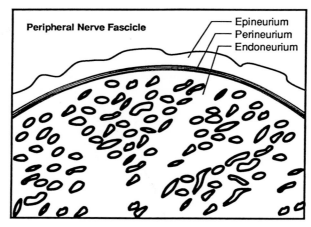

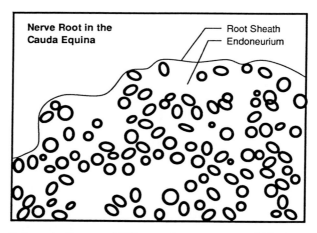

FIGURE 3. Schematic: Structural differences between nerves within the cauda equina and a peripheral nerve. Note that peripheral nerve fibers are located within the endoneurium, and the fascicles are surrounded by the perineurium, and outside this sheath is the epineurium, which is a connective tissue stroma located around and in between the fascicles of the nerve trunk. Nerve roots of the cauda equina, however, have no epineurium and essentially no perineurium, just a very thin root sheath.

subarachnoid space,[37,38] which might contribute to edema formation. The work of Schönström et al.[39] demonstrated that a decrease in the thecal sac diameter of between 11.1 and 10.6 mm at L3 and L4, respectively, produced a critical point at which compression of nerve roots occurred. This compression was thought to be responsible for a number of neurophysiological changes that may be categorized by the following: first, the biomechanics of nerve and nerve root injury; second, the intraneural blood flow alterations; third, increased vascular permeability leading to intraneural edema; fourth, effects on axonal transport; fifth, inflammation accompanied by demyelination; and the sixth, atrophy with wallerian degeneration followed by regeneration. Sunderland[4] has discussed the mechanics of peripheral nerves in detail. He points out that peripheral nerve *in vivo* are under some tension, a fact reflected by the phenomenon that nerves retract about 10–20% of their original length if cut. Intraneural blood flow is gradually impaired as the peripheral nerve is stretched to about 8% beyond *in vivo* strain; in this range, circulatory changes start to occur; intraneural blood flow ceases at about 15% beyond *in vivo* strain.[40]

Conflicting opinions exist regarding which tissue components of the peripheral nerve are responsible for its tensile properties. Sunderland[41] claims that the elasticity and tensile strength reside in the fascicular tissue, particularly in the perineurium. Haftek[42] claims that the elasticity of the nerve trunk depends primarily on the epineurium, less on the perineurium, and only slightly on interfascicular tissue.

The nerve roots in the thecal sac generally lack epineurium and perineurium, but under tensile loading exhibit both elasticity and tensile strength.[43] The ultimate load of the ventral motor spinal nerve roots from the thecal sac is from between 2 and 22 N and that for dorsal sensory nerve roots from the thecal sac is between 5 and 33 N.[4,43] The mechanical properties of a human spinal nerve root are different, depending upon its location within the central spinal canal and/or the lateral intervertebral foramina. It has been estimated that ultimate loads are approximately five times higher for foraminal segments of the spinal nerve roots than for the intrathecal portion of the same nerve roots under tensile loading.[44]

Information on the direct effects of nerve root pressure and axonal function is derived from peripheral nerve compression models. There is deformation of the nerve fibers, primarily at the edges of the compressed segment, and the nodes of Ranvier are displaced toward the noncompressed parts of the nerve.[45] Nodal displacement is followed by demyelination and conduction block; this is reversible, although some axonal loss and wallerian degeneration may occur.[455] Unmyelinated C-fibers are generally spared by this process, as compression primarily effects large myelinated fibers. However, severe compression may produce degeneration across the spectrum of fiber diameter types.

Nerve roots are not static structures. They move with relative freedom within the CSF and at each functional spinal unit relative to the surrounding tissues. It is this micromotion that allows the nerve root to maintain its mechanical properties and receive nutrition. Chronic irritation and subsequent fibrosis around nerve roots secondary to a herniated disc and/or stenosis can impair this movement and effect repeated injury to the nerve roots even during their attempted normal movements. Tissue irritation may in some ways be responsible for the various symptom complexes we encounter clinically.

Intraneural Blood Flow Alternations

Available evidence indicates that ischemia plays an important role in the clinical syndromes of nerve and nerve root compression. It is well known in cases of spinal stenosis, for which decompression surgeries are performed, that many patients can expect a significant clinical relief. Similar immediate relief is seen after removal of a herniated nucleus pulposus.[46–50] Hypothetically, nerve roots lacking a well-developed endoneurial blood-nerve barrier are more susceptible to compression injury than peripheral nerves, with increased risk of endoneurial edema formation.

Inflammation Edema and Demyelination

Autoimmune mechanisms have been implicated in inflammatory tissue reactions seen around degenerating discs.[51–53] It is these local inflammatory reactions in and around nerve roots in association with an intervertebral disc herniation that may be responsible for biochemical irritation from a mechanical stimulus.

Nerve Root Atrophy Degeneration and Regeneration

In spinal stenosis there is often a mixed lesion of the nerve roots. Atrophy, demyelination, and evidence of regeneration have all been documented.[54] Holts and Yates demonstrated that compression of roots or ganglia is associated with increased amounts of connective tissue around the Schwann cells, signs of axonal and myelin degeneration, and proliferation of Schwann cells. Obviously if cell death predominates, the potential for recovery of nerve function is limited. It is well known that more proximal lesions are associated with more profound degeneration of the cell body and lesions central to the dorsal root ganglion do not have a regenerative potential equivalent to that of lesions peripheral to the ganglion.[32,41] Therefore, lesions in the cauda equina may produce serious and less reversible neurologic injury than an analogous injury in the periphery. To summarize, compression may produce a series of events resulting from ischemia, inflammation, demyelination, and increased permeability, to various blood-borne and cerebral spinal fluid substances, with secondary endoneurial edema, degeneration, and regeneration of axons with chronic fibrosis. Thus, a degenerative spiral manifests itself as a syndrome that combines elements of functional loss and pain.

Neural Physiological Consequences of Nerve Injury

Nerve roots are not normally sensitive to mechanical stimulation. However, a nerve root at the site of chronic inflammation may produce radicular symptoms. This has been demonstrated in humans by placing ligatures or inflatable balloons around nerve roots at the time of surgery for a herniated disc and then mechanically stimulating the roots by traction and/or compression of the root postoperatively.[55,56] Howe and associates[57] in an experimental model demonstrated that compression of normal roots induces only brief discharges. However, roots that are chronically inflamed and demyelinated produced long discharges similar to the normal dorsal root ganglion. Burchiel and his colleagues have shown that neurons of the dorsal root ganglion also become spontaneously active after experiencing lesions of their peripheral processes.[58,59] Experimental compression of the dorsal root ganglion in rat induced edema, with increased tissue pressure in the ganglion.[24] Such edema can lead to fibrosis, altered histologic characteristics, and abnormal function in the compressed ganglion. One can speculate that this abnormal function may result in the abnormal sensitivity of the dorsal root ganglion. It has been shown that lesions of the peripheral nerve, dorsal root ganglion, and/or nerve roots themselves can result in generation of ectopic impulses identical to those described in neuromas.[60] Another mechanism that might cause continuing after pain after injury is mediated by the sympathetic nervous system. To date there are no well-documented cases of nerve root injury confined to the area within the spinal canal in which the pain was shown to be sympathetically maintained. Nonetheless, we do know that the sympathetic nervous system may play an important role in nerve injury and therefore should be considered in the analysis. One hypothesis is that sympathetically maintained pain results from the development of the alpha nerve receptors and nociceptive afferent fibers.[61]

CHEMICAL MEDIATION OF NOCICEPTION

As previously stated, pain originating in the lumbar spine typically arises from mechanical and/or chemical irritation of primary sensory neurons. The site of activation may involve the peripheral terminal endings of these neurons and tissues, such as muscles, joints, skin, periosteum, blood vessels, and meninges. Alternatively, it may involve a mechanical or chemical irritation to the dorsal root fiber or the soma within the dorsal root ganglion.[62] Some of the endogenous chemical substances, particularly inflammatory mediators, can excite or increase the excitability of primary sensory neurons or otherwise alter their local environment.

Nociceptors are the peripheral terminal endings of sensory neurons that are selectively responsive to potentially or overtly injurious stimuli that cause pain in humans and cause affective pain-like responses in animals.

CHEMICAL MEDIATORS OF PAIN

Non-neurogenic

A variety of endogenous chemicals are released from nonneural tissues, all of which have pain-producing capabilities. These include bradykinin, serotonin, histamine, acetylcholine, prostaglandins, E_1 and E_2, and leukotrienes.[62-64] Serotonin and bradykinin excite heat-sensitive or mechanosensitive C- or A-fiber nociceptive afferents innervating the skin, joints, skeletal, muscle and visceral organs.[64-74] There are various interactions among these chemicals and their physical stimuli as they affect nociceptor responses. Prostaglandins enhance the responses of C or A nociceptors in skin, joint, or muscle to heat, mechanical stimuli, or bradykinin.[65-78] Similarly, intradermal or subdermal injections of prostaglandin E_1 in humans produce mechanical tenderness and potentiate the pain from subdermal injections of bradykinin and the itch from histamine. Two other endogenous chemicals that have recently been shown to produce hyperalgesia are formed by the lipoxygenation of arachidonic acid: (1) dihydroxyeicosatetraenoic acid (diHETE), 15-lipoxygenase product, and (2) leukotriene B_4, a 5-lipoxygenase product. Leukotriene B_4 is a chemotaxin for polymorphonuclear leukocytes that accumulate at locations of inflammation to destroy antigens.[79] Leukotriene injected interdermally into the rat paw sensitizes C-nociceptors to mechanical stimuli and produces hyperalgesia. Further, this hyperalgesia is dependent upon the presence of polymorphonuclear leukocytes.[80] The hyperalgesia resulting from these substances is not blocked by nonsteroidal anti-inflammatory drugs that block the cyclo-oxgenation of arachidonic acid[81] (Fig. 4). Levine and associates[82] provided evidence that diHETE injected interdermally into the rat paw produces a hyperalgesia equivalent in maximal effect to that produced by leukotriene B_4, bradykinin, or prostaglandin E_2 (Fig. 5). Saal et al. have suggested phospholipase A_2 activity may be extremely important in the presence of a clinical radiculopathy associated with a herniated nucleus pulposus.[83]

Neurogenic Pain Mediators

For more than a decade a large number of primary afferent neurons have been known to produce neuropeptides such as substance P (SP).[84] These neuropeptides are produced within the dorsal root ganglion in cell bodies of primary afferent neurons and delivered by axonal transport to both the central and peripheral processes of neurons. Although SP from primary afferent neurons

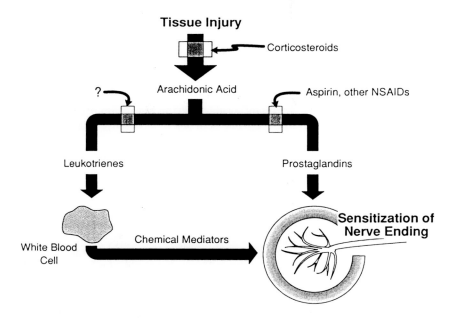

FIGURE 4. Diagram demonstrating that the leukotrienes, non-neurogenic mediators, are not affected by nonsteroidal anti-inflammatory agents but seem to be affected by steroids.

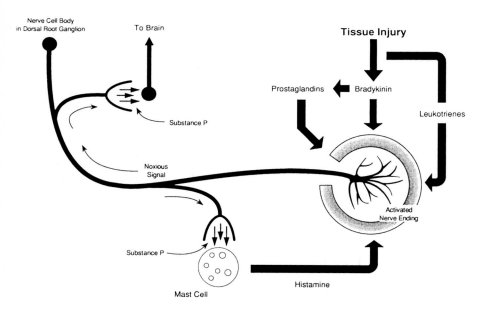

FIGURE 5. The interaction between peripheral tissue injury and repair and the central neurogenic components. This scheme demonstrates how neurogenic mediators can affect non-neurogenic mediators through the stimulation of mast cells by substance P.

has been demonstrated in response to intense electrical stimulation of peripheral nerves,[85] as has the excitatory effect of SP on ascending projection neurons,[86] it remains to be established whether SP (or any other neuropeptide within primary afferent neurons) is both necessary and sufficient as the chemical transmitter mediating nociception at the first synapse. This uncertainty stems from several sources. Capsaicin has been employed widely as a toxin for the reduction of peptides in primary afferent neurons. Studies using capasicin have attempted to discern the role of neuropeptides in primary afferent neurons and nociception. Its limitation is that it may not destroy peptides in myelinated primary afferent nerve fibers.[87-90] These residual myelinated peptidergic fibers may play an important role in nociception and, therefore, confound the interpretation of experiments in which capsaicin is used.

The number of neuropeptides now known to occur in primary afferent neurons has been steadily increasing. In addition to SP, somatostatin, cholecystokinin-like substance, vasoactive intestinal polypeptide, calcitonin gene-related peptide, gastrin-releasing peptide, dynorphin, enkephalin, and galanin are neuropeptides predominantly produced by primary afferent neurons.[91-102] Each of these peptides is likely to be produced by a biosynthetic precursor that may, through post-translational processing, give rise to additional biologically active peptides. Thus, the potential number of biologically active peptides produced by primary afferent neurons is high and confounds this simple examination of their role and/or roles in nociception. Anatomic studies of neuropeptides in the dorsal root ganglion cells have found these neurons to contain enzymes that, by their presence, implicate their substrates as playing a role in neurotransmission or neuromodulaton (for example, adenosine deaminase, which implicates purines, and fluoride-resistant acid phosphatase, whose substrate is unknown).[103] Neuropeptides are released from peripheral endings of nociceptive afferents as a result of noxious chemical or physical stimulation and can influence the inflammatory process.[104] Antidromatically induced release of neuropeptides by electrical stimulation of C-fibers can increase blood flow and vascular permeability. Substance P is believed to act directly on the blood vessels to produce plasma extravasation and indirectly to produce vascular dilatation by releasing histamine. Antihistamines and SP antigens block the flare induced by histamine; however, it seems that SP antagonists do not block the flare produced by capsaicin, suggesting that the final vasodilator is not histamine. Another candidate mediator is calcitonin gene-related peptide, which is a potent vasodilator and is co-localized with SP.[92]

Neuropeptides are also known to stimulate the release from mast cells of leukotrienes and other factors that attract and stimulate polymorphonuclear leukocytes and monocytes.[104] Certain pathologic conditions are accompanied by an increased SP; for example, increased SP is seen in peripheral nerves supplying arthritic joints and in cerebral spinal fluid of patients with low back pain and chronic arachnoiditis.[105] Substance P is released into joint tissues and stimulates proliferation of rheumatoid synovial sites and their release of prostaglandin E_2 and collagenase, thereby implicating this peptide in the pathogenesis of rheumatoid arthritis.[106] In addition, it has been demonstrated that VIP can cause a dose-dependent increase of bone resorption by a cAMP-dependent mechanism. Neuropeptides such as calcitonin gene-related peptide and SP can also contribute to the repair of injured tissue by stimulating the proliferation of smooth muscle cells and fibroblasts.[107]

Recently, it has been demonstrated that degeneration of the lumbar spine secondary to vibration, a known epidemiological cause of low back pain, may in part be related to neurogenic pain modulators.[2,28,108] Work designed to establish and develop animal-based experimental paradigms and techniques for studying degeneration of the components of the functional spinal unit has established that low frequency vibration causes changes in the amounts of SP and vasoactive intestinal peptide (VIP) in the dorsal root ganglion. The presence of these neuropeptides in the dorsal root ganglion, as well as in peripheral areas such as the disc annulus, facet joints, and blood plasma, suggests exciting possibilities for explaining chronic degeneration of the spinal motion segment.[28,108] Results from preliminary studies have motivated the development of a working model explaining chronic functional spinal unit degeneration that hypothesize causal links between environmental factors (e.g., vibration), and functional spinal unit degeneration mediated by biological events. The model is as follows: The release of neuropeptides from the dorsal root ganglion, induced by environmental and structural factors (i.e., vibrations), mediates a progressive degeneration of the functional spinal unit structures by stimulating the synthesis of inflammatory agents (e.g., prostaglandin E_2) and degradative enzymes (e.g., collagenase). The weakened functional spinal unit structures increase the susceptibility of the dorsal root ganglion to environmental factors, which, in turn, lowers the threshold necessary to stimulate neuropeptide activity, thereby creating a degenerative spiral (Fig. 6).

CENTRAL MODULATION OF PAIN

Finally, pain is not a one-way street. We are now beginning to formulate a better understanding of descending influences on pain perception and modulation. In the dorsal horn of the spinal cord, the site of the first synapse of pain pathways, is where neurotransmitters modulate nociceptive processing both pre- and postsynaptically. Both input from primary afferent neurons, as well as convergent, peptidergic input from local circuit neurons and descending bulbospinal neurons of the spinal cord and midbrain, affect responses made at the first synaptic junction.

A great deal of attention has been given to opioidergic neurons in the spinal cord because of their ability to inhibit nociceptive transmission. However, neurotensin, a non-opioid neuropeptide found in the spinal cord, also has inhibitory capacities.[109,110]

Neurons known to be peptidergic have been identified in the cerebral cortex and subthalamic, spinohypothalamic-telencephalic pathways. Surprisingly, however, the spinothalamic tract itself may not utilize neuropeptides for neurotransmission.

Families of endogenous, morphine-like, opioids have been described. Most familiar, of course, are the B-endorphins. Other less well known, but not less important, endogenous chemicals are dynorphins. These act at several different types of receptors. Endorphins typically act at the mu-receptors, whereas dynorphins have an affinity for the K-receptors. In the spinal cord the principal source of opioidlike peptides are the intrinsic dorsal horn neurons themselves. Most are local circuit interneurons.

We have now explored some very basic information about pain, its perception, and its modulations. The tunnel, however, remains dark and many questions are without answers. Investigations to find answers to basic questions about pain must continue in order to lead to a greater appreciation of mechanisms underlying this most elusive symptom.

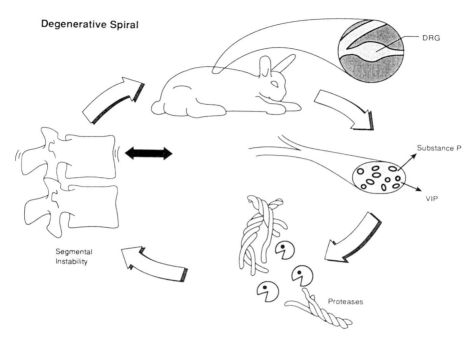

FIGURE 6.   "Degenerative spiral": The functional spinal unit may undergo degeneration as a result of the interaction of mechanical and chemical stimuli seen in an injured or environmentally stimulated functional spinal unit (Weinstein).

REFERENCES

1. Merskey H: Pain terms: A list with definitions and notes on usage. Recommended by the IASP Subcommittee on Taxonomy. Pain 6:249, 1979.
2. Frymoyer J: New Perspectives on Low Back Pain. A Workshop. Airlie Virginia, AAOS Publishers, May 1989.
3. Rydevik B, McLean WG, Sjöstrand J, et al: Blockage of axonal transport induced by acute, graded compression of the rabbit vagus nerve. J Neurol Neurosurg Psychiatry 43:690–6908, 1980.
4. Sunderland S: Nerve and nerve injuries. In Peripheral Sensory Mechanism, 2nd ed. New York, Churchill Livingstone, 1978.
5. Spencer DL, Irvin GS, Miller JA: Anatomy and significance of fixation of the lumbosacral nerve roots in sciatica. Spine 8:672–679, 1983.
6. Bogduk N, Twomey LT: Clinical Anatomy of the Lumbar Spine. Edinburgh, Churchill Livingstone, 1987.
7. Parke WW: Applied anatomy of the spine. In Rothman RH, Simeone F (eds): The Spine, 2nd ed. Philadelphia, WB Saunders, 1982.
8. Pedersen HE, Blunck CFJ, Gardner E: Anatomy of lumbosacral rami and meningeal branches of spinal nerves. J Bone Joint Surg 38A:377–391, 1956.
9. Hirsch C, Ingelmark B, Miller M: The anatomical basis for low back pain. Acta Orthop Scand 33:2, 1963.
10. Malinsky J: The ontogenetic development of nerve terminations in the intervertebral discs of man. Acta Anat 38:96, 1959.
11. Ralston HF, Miller MR, Kasahara M: Nerve endings in human fasciae, tendons, ligaments, periosteum, and joint synovial membrane. Anat Rec 136:137, 1960.
12. Jackson HC, Winkelman RK, Bickel WH: Nerve endings in the human lumbar spinal column and related structures. J Bone Joint Surg 48A:1271, 1966.
13. Wyke BD: The neurology of low back pain. In Jayson MIV (ed): The Lumbar Spine and Back Pain, 2nd ed. Kent, U.K., Pitman Medical Publishing, 1980, p 265.

14. Ikara C: A study of the mechanisms of low back pain. The neurohistochemical examination of disease. J Bone Joint Surg 36A:195, 1954.

15. Sherman MS: The nerves of bone. J Bone Joint Surg 45A:522, 1963.

16. Roofe PG: Innervation of the annulus fibrosus and posterior longitudinal ligament. Arch Neurol Psych 44:100, 1940.

17. Shinohara H: Lumbar disc lesion with special reference to the histological significance of nerve endings of the lumbar discs. J Jap Orthop Assoc 44:553–570, 1970.

18. Wall PD, Melzack R: Textbook of Pain. Edinburgh, Churchill Livingstone, 1984, pp 1–15.

19. Melzack R, Wall PD: Pain mechanisms: A new theory. Science 150:971–979, 1965.

20. Lindblom K, Rexed B: Spinal nerve injury in dorso-lateral protrusions of lumbar disks. J Neurosurg 5:413–432, 1948.

21. Lieberman AR: Sensory ganglia. In London DN (ed): The Peripheral Nerve. London, Chapman & Hall, 1976, pp 188–278.

22. Gibson SJ, Polak JM, Bloom SR, et al: The distribution of nine peptides in rat spinal cord with special emphasis on the substantia gelantinosa and on the area around the central canal (lamina X). J Comp Neurol 201:65–79, 1981.

23. Bergman L, Alexander L: Vascular supply of the spinal ganglia. Arch Neurol Psychiatry 46:761–782, 1941.

24. Rydevik BL, Myers RR, Powell HC: Tissue fluid pressure in the dorsal root ganglion: An experimental study on the effects of compression. Trans Orthop Res Soc 13:135, 1988; Spine 14(6):574–576, 1989.

25. Delamarter RB, Bohlman HH, Dodge LD, Biro D: Experimental lumbar spinal stenosis. J Bone Joint Surg 72A:110–120, 1990.

26. Dale H: Pharmacology and nerve-endings. Proc R Soc Med Ther 18:319–332, 1935.

27. Shantha TR, Evans JA: The relationship of epidural anesthesia to neural membranes and arachnoid villi. Anesthesiology 37(5):543–557, 1972.

28. Weinstein JN, Claverie W, Gibson S: The pain of discography. Spine 13:1344–1348, 1988.

29. Lundborg G, Myers R, Powell H: Nerve compression injury and increased endoneurial fluid pressure: A "miniature compartment syndrome." J Neurol Neurosurg Psychiatry 46:1119–1124, 1983.

30. Rydevik B, Nordborg C: Changes in nerve function and nerve fibre structure induced by acute, graded compression. J Neurol Neurosurg Psychiatry 43:1070–1082, 1980.

31. Rydevik B, Brown MD, Lundborg G: Pathoanatomy and pathophysiology of nerve root compression. Spine 9:7–15, 1984.

32. Sunderland S: Avulsion of nerve roots. In Vinken PJ, Bruyn GW (eds): Handbook of Clinical Neurology, Vol 25. Injuries of the Spine and Spinal Cord, Part I. New York, American Elsevier, 1975, pp 393–435.

33. Rydevik B, Lundborg G, Bagge U: Effects of graded compression on intraneural blood flow: An in vivo study on rabbit tibial nerve. J Hand Surg 6:3–12, 1981.

34. Dahlin LB, Rydevik B, Lundborg G: Pathophysiology of nerve entrapments and nerve compression injuries. In Hargens AR (ed): Tissue Nutrition and Viability. New York, Springer-Verlag, 1986, 135–160.

35. Gelfan S, Tarlov IM: Physiology of spinal cord, nerve root and peripheral nerve compression. Am J Physiol 185:217–229, 1956.

36. Sharpless SK: Susceptibility of spinal roots to compression block: The research status of spinal manipulative therapy. In Goldstein M (ed): NINCDS Monograph No. 15. Washington, DC, Government Printing Office, 1975, pp 155–161.

37. Arvidson B: Distribution of intravenously injected protein tracers in peripheral ganglia of adult mice. Exp Neurol 63:388, 1979.

38. Olsson Y: The involvement of vasa nervorum in disease of peripheral nerves. In Vinken PS, Bruyn GW (eds): Handbook of Clinical Neurology, Vol 12. Vascular Disease of the Nervous System, Part 2. New York, American Elsevier, 1972, pp 644–664.

39. Shönström N, Bolender NF, Spengler DM, et al: Pressure changes within the cauda equina following constriction of the dural sac: An in vitro experimental study. Spine 9:604–607, 1984.

40. Lundborg G, Rydevik B: Effects of stretching the tibial nerve of the rabbit: A preliminary study of the intraneural circulation and the barrier function of the perineurium. J Bone Joint Surg 55B:390–401, 1973.

41. Sunderland S, Bradley KC: Stress-strain phenomena in human peripheral nerve trunks. Brain 84:102–119, 1961.

42. Haftek J: Stretch injury of peripheral nerve: Acute effects of stretching on rabbit nerve. J Bone Joint Surg 52B:354–365, 1970.

43. Sunderland S, Bradley KC: Stress-strain phenomena in human spinal nerve roots. Brain 84:120–124, 1984.
44. Kwan MK, Rydevik BL, Brown R, et al: Selected biomechanical assessment of lumbosacral spinal nerve roots. Presented at the Meeting of the International Society for the Study of the Lumbar Spine, Miami, Florida, April 1988.
45. Ochta J, Fowler TJ, Gilliatt RW: Anatomical changes in peripheral nerves compressed by a pneumatic tourniquet. J Anat 113:433–455, 1972.
46. Evans JG: Neurogenic intermittent claudication. Br Med J 2:985–987, 1964.
47. Wilson CB, Ehni G, Grollmus J: Neurogenic intermittent claudication. Clin Neurosurg 18:62–85, 1971.
48. Wiltse LL, Kirkaldy-Willis WH, McIvor GW: The treatment of spinal stenosis. Clin Orthop 115:83–91, 1976.
49. Epstein BS, Epstein JA, Jones MD: Lumbar spinal stenosis. Radiol Clin North Am 15:117–139, 1977.
50. Rydevik B, Lundborg G, Nordborg C: Intraneural tissue reactions induced by internal neurolysis: An experimental study on the blood-nerve barrier, connective tissues and nerve fibres of rabbit tibial nerve. Scand J Plast Reconst Surg 10:3–8, 1976.
51. Bobechko WP, Hirsch C: Auto-immune response to nucleus pulposus in the rabbit. J Bone Joint Surg 47B:574–580, 1965.
52. Gertzbein SD, Tile M, Gross A, et al: Autoimmunity in degenerative disc disease of the lumbar spine. Orthop Clin North Am 6:67–73, 1975.
53. McCarron RF, Wimpee MW, Hudkins PG, et al: The inflammatory effect of nucleus pulposus: A possible element in the pathogenesis of low back pain. Spine 12:760–764, 1987.
54. Watanabe R, Parke WW: Vascular and neural pathology of lumbosacral spinal stenosis. J Neurosurg 65:64–70, 1986.
55. Macnab I: The mechanism of spondylogenic pain. In Hirsch C, Zotterman Y (eds): Cervical Pain. Oxford, Pergamon Press, 1972, pp 88–95.
56. Smyth MJ, Wright V: Sciatica and the intervertebral disc: An experimental study. J Bone Joint Surg 40A:1401–1418, 1958.
57. Howe JF, Loeser JD, Calvin WH: Mechanosensitivity of dorsal root ganglia and chronically injured axons: A physiological basis for the radicular pain of nerve root compression. Pain 3:25–41, 1977.
58. Burchiel KJ: Effects of electrical and mechanical stimulation on two foci of spontaneous activity which develop in primary afferent neurons after peripheral axotomy. Pain 85:257–272, 1984.
59. Wall PD, Devor M: Sensory afferent impulses originate from dorsal root ganglia and chronically injured axons: A physiological basis for the radicular pain of nerve root compression. Pain 17:321–339, 1983.
60. Nordin M, Nyström B, Wallin U, et al: Ectopic sensory discharges and paresthesias in patients with disorders of peripheral nerves, dorsal roots and dorsal columns. Pain 20:231–245, 1984.
61. Campbell JN, Raja SN, Meyer RA: Painful sequelae of nerve injury. In Dubner R, Gebhart GF, Bond MR (eds): Pain Research and Clinical Management. Amsterdam, Elsevier (in press).
62. Wyke B: Receptor systems in lumbosacral tissues in relation to the production of low back pain. In White AA III, Gordon SL (eds): American Academy of Orthopaedic Surgeons Symposium on Idiopathic Low Back Pain. St. Louis, CV Mosby, 1982, pp 97–107.
63. Ferreira SH: Prostaglandins, aspirin-like drugs and analgesia. Nature (New Biol) 240:200–230, 1972.
64. Kanaka R, Schaible HG, Schmidt RF: Activation of fine articular afferent units by bradykinin. Brain Res 327:81–90, 1985.
65. Handwerker HO: Influences of algogenic substances and prostaglandins on the discharges of unmyelinated cutaneous nerve fibers identified as nociceptors. In Bionca JJ, Fessard D (eds): Advances in Pain Research and Therapy. New York, Raven Press, 1976.
66. Beck PW, Handwerker HO: Bradykinin and serotonin effects of various types of cutaneous nerve fibres. Pflügers Arch 347:209–22, 1974.
67. Chahl LA, Iggo A: The effects of bradykinin and prostaglandin E_1 on rat cutaneous afferent nerve activity. Br J Pharmacol 59:343–3447, 1977.
68. Khan AA, Raja SN, Campbell JN, et al: Bradykinin sensitizes nociceptors to heat stimuli. Soc Neurosci Abst 12:219, 1986.
69. Szolcsanyi J: Selective responsiveness of polymodal nociceptors of the rabbit ear to capasicin, bradykinin and ultra-violet irradiation. J Physiol 388:9–23, 1987.
70. Franz M, Mense S: Muscle receptors with Group IV afferent fibres responding to application of bradykinin. Brain Res 91:369–383, 1975.

71. Hiss E, Mense S: Evidence for the existence of different receptor sites for algesic agents at the endings of muscular Group IV afferent units. Pflügers Arch 361:1441–146, 1976.

72. Mense S: Nervous outflow from skeletal muscle following chemical noxious stimulation. J Physiol 167:75–88, 1977.

73. Mense S, Schmidt RF: Activation of Group IV afferent units from muscle by algesic agents. Brain Res 72:305–310, 1974.

74. Mense S: Sensitization of Group IV muscle receptors to bradykinin by 5-hydroxytrypamine and prostaglandin E_2. Brain Res 225:95–105, 1981.

75. Martin HA, Basbaum AI, Kwiat GC, et al: Leukotriene and prostaglandin sensitization of cutaneous high-threshold C- and A-delta mechanonociceptors in the hairy skin of rat hindlimbs. Neuroscience 22:651–659, 1987.

76. Reeh PW: Sensory receptors in a mammalian skin-nerve in vitro preparation. Prog Brain Res (in press).

77. Pateromichelakis S, Rood JP: Prostaglandin E_1-induced sensitization of A-δ moderate pressure mechanoreceptors. Brain Res 232:89–96, 1982.

78. Pateromichelakis S, Rood JP: Prostaglandin E_2 increases mechanically evoked potentials in the peripheral nerve. Experientia 37:282–284, 1981.

79. Ford-Hutchinson AW, Brady MA, Doig MV, et al: Leukotriene B, a potent chemokinetic and aggregating substance released from polymorphonuclear leukocytes. Nature 286:264–265, 1980.

80. Kumazawa T, Mizumura K: The polymodal receptors in the testes of dog. Brain Res 139:553–5558, 1977.

81. Levine JD, Gooding J, Donatoni P, et al: The role of the polymorphonuclear leukocyte in hyperalgesia. J Neurosci 5:3025–3029, 1985.

82. Levine JD, Lam D, Taiwo YO, et al: Hyperalgesic properties of 15-lipooxygenase products of arachidonic acid. Proc Natl Acad Sci USA 83:5331–5334, 1986.

83. Saal JS, Dobrow R, Saal JA, et al: Biochemical evidence of inflammation. Presented to International Society for the Study of the Lumbar Spine, Kyoto, Japan, May 1989.

84. Hökflet T, Elde R, Johannson O, et al: Immunohistochemical evidence for separate populations of somatostatin-containing and substance P-containing primary afferent neurons in the rat. Neuroscience 1:131–136, 1976.

85. Yaksh TL, Jessell TM, Gamse R, et al: Intrathecal morphine inhibits substance P release from mammalian spinal cord in vivo. Nature 286:155–157, 1980.

86. Willcockson WS, Chung JM, Hori Y, et al: Effects of iontophoretically released peptides on primate spinothalamic tract cells. J Neurosci 4:741–750, 1984.

87. Ruda MA, Bennett GJ, Dubner R: Neurochemistry and neural circuitry in the dorsal horn. Prog Brain Res 66:219–268, 1986.

88. Tuchscherer MM, Seybold VS: Immunohistochemical studies of substance P, cholecystokinin-octapeptide and somatostatin in dorsal root ganglia of the rat. Neuroscience 14:593–605, 1985.

89. Tuchscherer MM, Knox C, Seybold VS: Substance P and cholecystokinin-like immunoreactive varicosities in somatosensory and autonomic regions of the rat spinal cord: A quantitative study of coexistence. J Neurosci 7:3984–3995, 1987.

90. Tuchscherer MM, Seybold VS: A quantitative study of the coexistence of peptides in the varicosities within the superficial laminae of the dorsal horn of the rat spinal cord. J Neurosci (in press).

91. Wiesenfeld-Hallin Z, Hökfelt T, Lundberg JM, et al: Immunoreactive calcitonin gene-related peptide and substance P coexist in sensory neurons to the spinal cord and interact in spinal behavioral responses of the rat. Neurosci Lett 52:199–204, 1984.

92. Lee Y, Takami K, Kawai Y, et al: Distribution of calcitonin gene-related peptide in rat peripheral nervous system with reference to its coexistence with substance P. Neuroscience 15:1227–1237, 1985.

93. Dalsgaard C-J, Vincent SR, Hökfelt T, et al: Coexistence of cholecystokinin- and substance P-like peptides in neurons of the dorsal root ganglia of the rat. Neurosci Lett 33:159–163, 1982.

94. Franco-Cereceda A, Henke H, Lundberg JM, et al: Calcitonin gene-related peptide (CGRP) in capsaicin-sensitive substance P-immunoreactive sensory neurons in animals and man: Distribution and release by capsaicin. Peptides 8:399–410, 1987.

95. Fuxe K, Agnati LF, McDonald T, et al: Immunohistochemical indications of gastrin releasing peptide-bombesin-like immunoreactivity in the nervous system of the rat: Codistribution with substance P-like immunoreactive nerve terminal systems and coexistence with substance P-like immunoreactivity in dorsal root ganglion cell bodies. Neurosci Lett 37:17–22, 1983.

96. Gibbins IL, Furness JB, Costa M, et al: Co-localization of calcitonin gene-related peptide-like immunoreactivity with substance P in cutaneous, vascular and visceral sensory neurons of guinea pigs. Neurosci Lett 57:125–130, 1985.

97. Gibbins IL, Furness JB, Costa M: Pathway-specific patterns of the co-existence of substance P, calcitonin gene-related peptide, cholecystokinin and dynorphin in neurons of the dorsal root ganglia of the guinea pig. Cell Tissue Res 148:417–437, 1987.

98. Gibson SJ, Polak JM, Bloom SR, et al: Calcitonin gene-related peptide immunoreactivity in the spinal cord of man and of eight other species. J Neurosci 4:3101–3111, 1984.

99. Leah JD, Cameron AA, Kell WL, et al: Coexistence of peptide immunoreactivity in sensory neurons of the cat. Neuroscience 16:683–690, 1985.

100. Lundberg JM, Franco-Cereceda A, Hua A, et al: Co-existence of substance P and calcitonin gene-related peptide-like immunoreactivities in sensory nerves in relation to cardiovascular and bronchoconstrictor effects of capsaicin. Eur J Pharmacol 108:315–319, 1985.

101. O'Donohue TL, Massari VJ, Pazoles CJ, et al: A role for bombesin in sensory processing in the spinal cord. J Neurosci 4:2956–2962, 1984.

102. Panula P, Hadjiconstantinou M, Yang H-YT, et al: Immunohistochemical localization of bombesin gastrin-releasing peptide and substance P in primary sensory neurons. J Neurosci 3:2021–2129, 1983.

103. Nagy JI, Daddona PE: Anatomical and cytochemical relationships of adenosine deaminase-containing primary afferent neurons in the rat. Neuroscience 15:799–813, 1985.

104. Payan DG, McGillis JP, Goetzl EJ: Neuroimmunology. Adv Immunol 39:299–323, 1986.

105. Howe JF, Calvin WH, Losser JD: Impulses reflected from dorsal root ganglia and from focal nerve injuries. Brain Res 116:139–144, 1900.

106. Lotz M, Carson DA, Vaughan JH: Substance P activation of rheumatoid synoviocytes: Neural pathway in pathogenesis of arthritis. Science 235:893–895, 1987.

107. Payan DG, McGillis JP, Renold FK: Neuropeptide modulation of leukocyte function. Ann NY Acad Sci 496:182–191, 1987.

108. Weinstein JN, Pope M, Schmidt R, Seroussi R: Neuropharmacologic effects of vibration on the dorsal root ganglion: An animal model. Spine 13:521–525, 1988.

109. Ruda MA, Coffield J, Dubner R: Demonstration of postsynaptic opioid modulation of thalamic projection neurons by the combined techniques of retrograde horesradish peroxidase and enkephalin immunocytochemistry. J Neurosci 4:2117–2132, 1984.

110. Seybold VS, Elde RP: Neurotensin immunoreactivity in the superficial laminae of the dorsal horn of the rat: I. Light microscopic studies of cell bodies and proximal deformities. J Comp Neurol 105:89–100, 1982.

RICHARD J. HERZOG, MD

STATE OF THE ART IMAGING STUDIES OF SPINAL DISORDERS

From the NeuroSkeletal
  Imaging Center
Daly City, California

Reprint requests to:
Richard J, Herzog, MD
Director, NeuroSkeletal Imaging
  Center
1850 Sullivan Avenue, Suite 110
Daly City, CA 94015

In all fields of medicine, therapeutic success is directly dependent upon the accuracy of diagnosis. In the process of evaluating a patient presenting with spinal pain or neural dysfunction, radiologic diagnostic studies are frequently needed to clarify the cause of the patient's symptoms. Plain film evaluation of the spinal column is frequently the first diagnostic examination ordered in the evaluation of suspected spinal disease, but due to its lack of sensitivity and specificity, the information obtained from radiographs is frequently limited.[52] Plain x-rays may be of benefit when evaluating spinal morphometry, chronic degenerative changes of the discovertebral joints, spondylolysis, spondylolisthesis, post-traumatic deformation, spinal infection, and evidence of metastatic disease. Unfortunately, abnormalities on plain x-rays are frequently detected relatively late in the natural history of most spinal disorders. Radiographic evaluation may be helpful in directing the choice of which advanced diagnostic imaging study should be ordered if additional clinical information is required.

Many fields of medicine have recently witnessed a rapid change in the application of new technologies to their diagnostic armamentarium. The recent advances in spinal imaging have been meteoric, and, as a result, the complexity of the imaging technologies has surpassed the understanding of many clinicians trying to utilize them.[15,76,148,155,156] This is particularly true for the two most advanced diagnostic exams currently performed in the evaluation of spinal disease, high resolution multiplanar computed tomography (CT/MPR) and magnetic resonance imaging (MRI).

The challenge in spinal imaging is not just to optimize the technical quality of imaging procedures, but also to maximize the information obtained from these diagnostic examinations. The purpose of this chapter is initially to discuss the basic physics and imaging protocols of CT/MPR and MRI, followed by a section on the clinical application of these two imaging procedures. Neither examination elucidates all the facets of spinal pathomorphology, and thus a diagnostic algorithm is needed to determine which procedure will provide the maximum information in different clinical settings. In many imaging centers, MRI has quickly become the primary imaging modality in the evaluation of spinal dysfunction,[9,103] even though there have been few rigorous, prospective, controlled comparative studies to evaluate the true diagnostic efficacy of MRI examinations.[32] My experience imaging the spine for the evaluation of spinal disorders includes both high-field strength (1.5 tesla) and mid-field strength (0.4 tesla) MRI systems and the performance of over 15,000 CT/MPR examinations.

PHYSICS AND TECHNIQUE

An image of an object may be defined as a graphical representation of the spatial distribution of one or more of its properties.[94] In a CT examination, an x-ray source is employed to generate cross-sectional images. CT images are representations of differential x-ray attenuation by tissue. This attenuation is determined by the tissue's electron density. Spatial and contrast resolution are dependent on the energy of the x-ray source, slice thickness, field of view, and scanning matrix. A variety of pre- and post-processing software programs are available to optimize the evaluation of soft tissue or osseous structures.[56,183] To obtain a high-resolution multiplanar CT study, it is necessary to utilize thin (1.5 mm) contiguous sections in the cervical spine and overlapping sections (5 mm thick with a 2 mm overlap) in the lumbar spine in order to create optimal computer-generated sagittal and coronal reconstructed images.[59,60] The diagnostic quality of a CT/MPR examination is highly dependent on patient immobility to prevent misregistration artifacts. An entire CT/MPR study can currently be performed in 20–25 minutes, and, therefore, it is usually not difficult for a patient to maintain a single position. With current rapid scanning techniques, patient x-ray exposure has been significantly reduced, but still the risk of radiation exposure must be considered when ordering an examination.

Whereas an image created with an x-ray source is determined by the electron density of the tissue being evaluated, MR images are a construct of totally different physical properties of tissue. If a nucleus of an atom contains either unpaired protons or neutrons, it will have a net spin and angular momentum.[25] Each spinning nucleus is surrounded by a magnetic field and can be thought of as a small bar magnet or dipole, with a north and south pole. If the body is placed in a static external magnetic field, i.e., the MR magnet, the normal random position of the nuclear dipoles in the body will be altered, and they will align themselves along the vector of the externally applied magnetic field. A magnetization vector of the tissue will be created that is the sum of the dipoles oriented in the same direction as the applied static magnetic field. When the spinning nuclei are aligned in the external magnetic field, they also precess (wobble) around the axis of the applied magnetic field. The frequency of this nuclear precession is called its resonant frequency and is proportional to the strength of the external magnetic field. At present, virtually all clinical MR imaging is performed by imaging hydrogen nuclei (proton imaging). Hydrogen is an ideal atom for imaging, being the most abundant resonant nucleus in soft tissues and providing a strong MR signal.[73]

To create an MR image, radio waves of a specific radio frequency (RF) are pulsed into the body, which induce the transition of a fraction of the spinning protons from their equilibrium state into a higher energy state. With the termination of the RF pulse, the excited nuclei release energy and return to their lower energy state. This characteristic absorption and release of energy is called nuclear magnetic resonance. The transition between energy states is necessary for the construction of an MR image.

The process of returning from the excited to the equilibrium state is called relaxation and is characterized by two independent time constants, T1 and T2. The T1 (longitudinal relaxation time) reflects the time required for excited protons to return to their equilibrium state. When the hydrogen nucleus is excited by the application of an RF pulse, in addition to changing to a higher energy state the initially random precession of the nuclei prior to excitation will become coherent (in phase) after excitation. This results in a magnetization vector perpendicular (transverse) to the external magnetic field that can be directly measured by a receiver coil. With the termination of the RF pulse, there is rapid loss of coherence of the precessing nuclei, and the T2 (transverse relaxation time) is the time reflecting the loss of the transverse magnetization.

T1 and T2 relaxation are intrinsic physical properties of tissue. The MR signal intensity is mainly dependent on the T1, T2, and proton-density (number of mobile hydrogen ions) of the tissue being evaluated. Flow also affects the signal intensity generated by body fluids. In order to obtain an anatomic image, spatial encoding of the energy released by the excited protons must be performed in three anatomic planes. This is accomplished by creating small-gradient magnetic fields within the larger static applied field. There are excellent texts that describe this process in detail.[19,116]

The methods for obtaining MR data are designated pulse sequences. Spin-echo (SE) and gradient echo (GE) are currently the pulse sequences most often employed. The spin-echo pulse sequence is probably the most commonly used MRI sequence, and the images created are dependent upon several scanning parameters. The repetition time (TR), the time between RF pulses, and the echo time (TE), the time between the application of the RF pulse and the time of recording the MR signal, are determined prior to acquiring the image. By varying the scanning parameters (TR and TE), the relative contributions of the T1, T2, and proton-density of the tissue will determine image contrast.[16] A T1-weighted image, which emphasizes the T1 properties of the tissue, is produced with a short TR (400–600 ms) and a short TE (15–30 ms). T1-weighted images are ideal for evaluating structures containing fat, subacute or chronic hemorrhage, or proteinaceous fluid, since these materials have a short T1 and yield a high signal on T1-weighted sequences. T1-weighted images, frequently thought of as fat images, are excellent in the delineation of anatomic structures. An MR image produced with a long TR (1500–2000 ms) and a short TE (15–30 ms) is referred to as a proton-density or spin-density weighted image, and the signal intensity reflects the absolute number of mobile hydrogen ions in the tissue. A T2-weighted sequence, which emphasizes the T2 properties of tissue, requires a long TR (1500–3000 ms) and a long TE (60–120 ms). The signal intensity on T2-weighted images is related to the state of hydration of the tissue. Any tissue rich in free or extracellular water, e.g., cerebrospinal fluid, cysts, necrotic tissue, fluid collections, intervertebral discs, and neoplasms, will demonstrate increased signal intensity on T2-weighted sequences. Mineral rich tissue, e.g., bone, contains few mobile protons and consequently demonstrates very low signal intensity on all pulse sequences. Gas, containing no mobile hydrogen ions, generates no MR signal.

In addition to signal intensity, tissue and organ configuration must be evaluated to detect pathologic changes. Spatial resolution, the ability to delineate fine detail, is determined by slice thickness, field of view (FOV), and the size of the acquisition and display matrices. Ideally, when imaging small structures, thin sections with a large matrix (256 × 256 or 512 × 512) should be utilized, but MRI like CT is affected by signal-to-noise constraints, and image degradation may result from low signal-to-noise ratios. Improved spatial resolution on MRI evaluations can be achieved employing surface coils, with their higher signal-to-noise ratio, but at the cost of a smaller field of view.[88]

As in all imaging procedures, artifacts are a source of image degradation in MRI studies, resulting in significant loss of diagnostic information.[7,9,166] Motion artifacts are the most common cause of image degradation, and unlike CT, with which patient motion results in degradation of a single image, movement during MRI scanning will cause degradation of all images in a sequence. In order to decrease scan time, new fast-scanning methods have been developed, gradient echo imaging being the one most frequently utilized.[17,172] The information obtained from gradient echo studies is different from standard T1- and T2-weighted sequences, and at this time it cannot be considered a simple replacement for a standard sequence.

IMAGING PROTOCOLS

CT/MPR Protocols

When performing a CT/MPR study, there are only a few choices that are necessary at the time of image acquisition to produce an excellent multiplanar examination. On the routine evaluation of the cervical spine, contiguous 1.5-mm thick sections are obtained from the pedicle of C3 or C4 to the pedicle of C7. Thin sections are necessary in the delineation of normal anatomy and pathologic changes in the cervical spine (Fig. 1). In the thoracic spine, contiguous 3-mm thick sections are obtained in the area of interest. Either four or five disc levels can be evaluated on a single study. In the lumbar spine, the routine examination includes overlapping 5-mm thick sections obtained at 3-mm intervals from the pedicle of L3 through the L5–S1 disc level (Fig. 2). After acquiring the initial axial images, computer generated contiguous sagittal and coronal images are created with a spacing of 1.5 mm between images in the cervical examination and 3 mm in the thoracic and lumbar examinations. To produce a complete CT/MPR study, it is mandatory that contiguous sagittal and coronal reformations be obtained to evaluate the spine in complementary orthogonal planes.[59] All images are photographed twice to optimally delineate soft tissue and osseous contrast. The strength of CT/MPR resides in its excellent delineation of osseous structures, and its main limitations are radiation exposure, slightly restricted field of view, and poor delineation of intrathecal anatomy and pathology.

MRI Protocols

In contrast to the CT/MPR evaluation, MRI is an operator-intensive imaging study with multiple parameters, e.g., TR, TE, number of excitations

(NEX), slice thickness, and matrix size, all of which are determined at the time of image acquisition.[16] Technical considerations to limit various artifacts must also be specified for each sequence. With the wide variety of tissue types evaluated in spinal MR imaging, the standard examination includes T1-weighted, proton-density, and T2-weighted sequences.[9] In addition, gradient echo sequences are frequently used in the evaluation of the cervical spine.[119]

The MRI examination must be tailored for the unique anatomy of the different parts of the spinal column. It is often tempting to shorten an imaging study when trying to answer a specific clinical question. In the evaluation of spinal disease, clinical symptoms and physical signs of neural dysfunction may not be easily localized to a specific motion segment,[2,90] and they can also be elicited by a variety of pathologic processes. For these reasons, it is critical that in each spinal region studied, all spinal and paraspinal anatomy must be completely examined and optimally displayed using sagittal, axial, and, when appropriate, additional nonorthogonal imaging sequences.

Prior to undergoing the MRI examination, each patient must be carefully questioned to determine if there are any contraindications to performing the study. Absolute contraindications include ferromagnetic cerebral aneurysm clips; cardiac pacemakers, which may become dysfunctional in high magnetic fields[127]; metallic foreign bodies in the orbit; and ferromagnetic cochlear implants. Pregnancy, recent cardiac or vascular surgery, transcutaneous electrical nerve stimulators, and severe claustrophobia are relative contraindications that must be handled on an individual basis to determine whether the benefit of a study outweighs the risk. Artifacts can be expected from a variety of metallic instrumentation devices[154] and from metallic particles in the body from previous trauma or surgery.[74] It is difficult to predict the degree of image degradation from metallic devices, and frequently an MRI study will be helpful even in patients with spinal instrumentation.

Cervical Spine Protocols

Due to the complex geometry and small size of the anatomic components of the cervical spine, imaging with high resolution surface coils is required. Thin section (3–3.5 mm) imaging with a small interslice gap in both axial and sagittal planes is necessary to delineate the normal neural structures in the spinal central and intervertebral canals (Fig. 3). The routine exam of the cervical spine includes both T1- and T2-weighted sequences to adequately evaluate all spinal and paraspinal anatomy.[105,129,168] The sagittal T1-weighted sequence covering an area from the cervicomedullary junction to the cervicothoracic junction provides an excellent survey of the vertebral bodies, intervertebral discs, spinal cord, thecal sac, and posterior elements. Axial T1-weighted images provide an excellent evaluation of spinal cord morphology, intrathecal nerve root anatomy, vertebral bodies, posterior elements, intervertebral canals, and paraspinal soft tissues. The main limitation of the T1-weighted sequence is due to the lack of MR signal from the vertebral body cortex, the posterior annular-posterior longitudinal ligament complex, and the cerebrospinal fluid in the adjacent thecal sac resulting in poor contrast differentiation among these structures.[123] This makes evaluation of small disc herniations, chondro-osseous spurs, and hypertrophied or calcified ligaments extremely difficult. To achieve a contrast difference between the posterior margin of the discovertebral joint and the thecal sac, either a cardiac-gated or flow-compensated T2-weighted sequence or a gradient

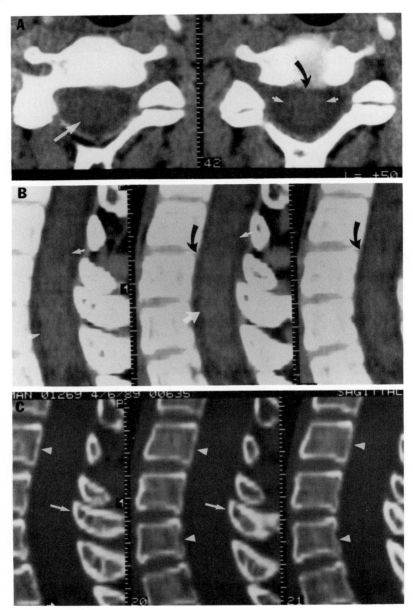

FIGURE 1. **Normal cervical spine anatomy**—CT/MPR. On the axial *(A)* and sagittal *(B)* images, the spinal cord (white arrows) is delineated along with the posterior margin of the disc (black arrow). The images have been photographed to optimize soft tissue resolution. The sagittal images through the midline *(C)* and the facet joints *(D) (see opposite page)* and the coronal images *(E)* have been photographed to evaluate optimally the osseous structures. There is excellent delineation of the vertebral bodies (white arrowheads), laminae (white arrows), facet joints (curved black arrows), and the intervertebral canals (curved white arrows).

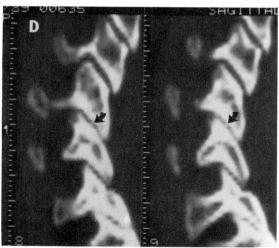

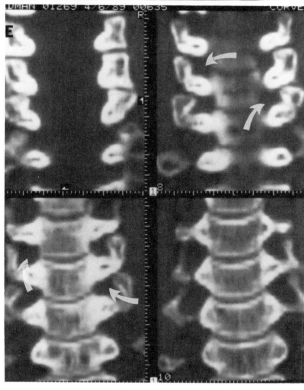

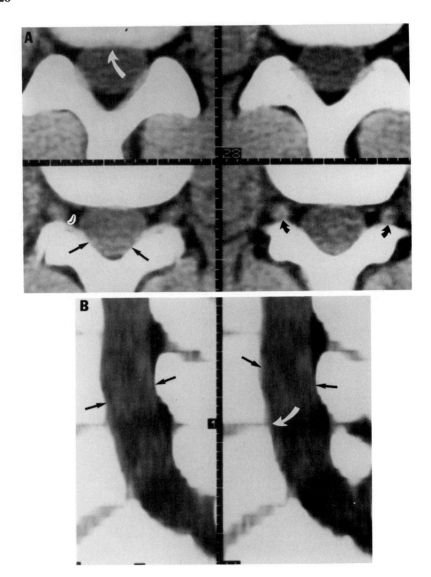

FIGURE 2. **Normal lumbar spine anatomy**—CT/MPR. On the axial *(A)* and sagittal *(B)* images, there is excellent delineation of the thecal sac (straight black arrows), dorsal root ganglia (curved black arrows) in the intervertebral canals, and the posterior margin of the discovertebral joints (curved white arrows). *(Figure continued.)*

echo sequence can be performed.[43,119] On both of these sequences, cerebrospinal fluid will generate high signal intensity, creating a CSF myelographic effect. This provides an excellent CSF-extradural interface and delineation of the spinal cord. Gradient echo sequences are helpful in the evaluation of extradural disease but not as a primary tool in the evaluation of spinal cord pathology or vertebral

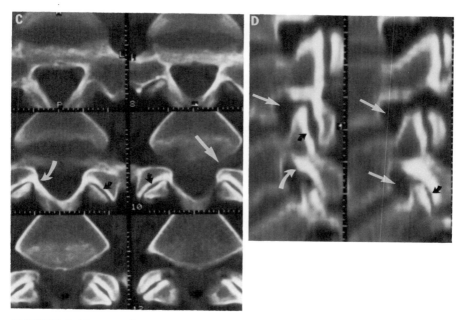

FIGURE 2 *(Continued).* On the axial *(C)* and sagittal *(D)* images, there is excellent delineation of the facet joints (curved black arrows). The intervertebral canals (straight white arrows) are optimally demonstrated on the sagittal images.

body marrow disease. Additional pulse sequences helpful in the evaluation of the cervical spine include oblique sequences through the intervertebral canals[72] and multiple-angled sections through the disc spaces.[138] Coronal sequences are helpful in the evaluation of spinal cord pathology, extradural masses, paraspinal pathology, and vertebral body malalignment or deformation.

Thoracic Spine Protocols

The initial sequence of a thoracic examination should include a sagittal T1-weighted localizer sequence that covers the entire cervical spine and cervicothoracic junction. This sequence provides the best reference for accurately numbering thoracic vertebral bodies and may also occasionally allow the detection of cervical spine disease presenting as thoracic neural dysfunction. The initial sequence evaluating the thoracic spine should be a sagittal T1-weighted localizer that includes the area from the cervicothoracic junction to the conus medullaris. This is followed by high-resolution sagittal T1 and multiecho T2-weighted sequences[102, 144, 180] (Fig. 4). A surface coil is employed to achieve high spatial resolution, and the field of view of these coils is usually adequate to evaluate the region from T1 or T2 to approximately T10 or T11. After the completion of the sagittal sequences, the examination should be reviewed by a radiologist to determine whether additional axial sequences are needed. These are obtained when a pathologic process is identified or if the patient's symptoms suggest a specific location of a disease process, even though this area appears normal on the initial sagittal images. This is particularly true in the evaluation of the intervertebral canals, paravertebral soft tissues, and posterior elements of the vertebrae, which are not

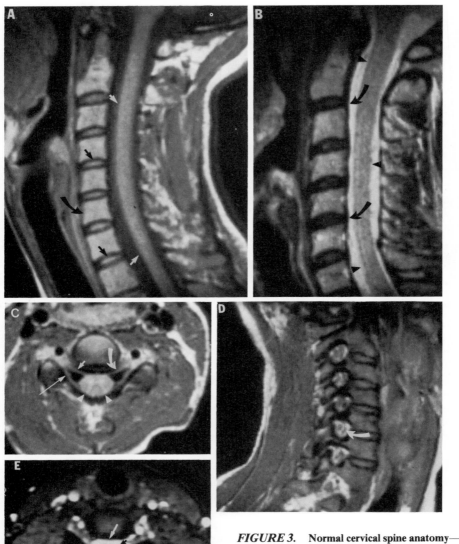

FIGURE 3. **Normal cervical spine anatomy—**
MRI. On the sagittal T1-weighted image *(A)*,
there is excellent anatomic delineation of the
vertebral bodies (curved black arrows), intervertebral discs (straight black arrows), and spinal cord
(white arrows). On the sagittal cardiac gated T2-
weighted image *(B)*, a myelographic effect is created
by the increased signal intensity in the cerebrospinal
fluid. There is an excellent interface between the posterior margin of the discovertebral joints (curved
black arrows) and the cerebrospinal fluid, and excellent delineation of the spinal cord (black
arrowheads). On the axial T1-weighted image *(C)*, there is excellent delineation of the spinal cord
(white arrowheads), ventral (short white arrow), and dorsal (long white arrow) nerve roots, and the
intervertebral canals (curved white arrow). On the oblique T1-weighted image *(D)*, the fat in the
intervertebral canals outlines the neural (curved arrow) and vascular structures. On the axial gradient
echo image *(E)*, the high signal intensity of the CSF produces excellent contrast for the delineation
of the spinal cord (black arrow) and the posterior margin of the discovertebral joint (white arrow).

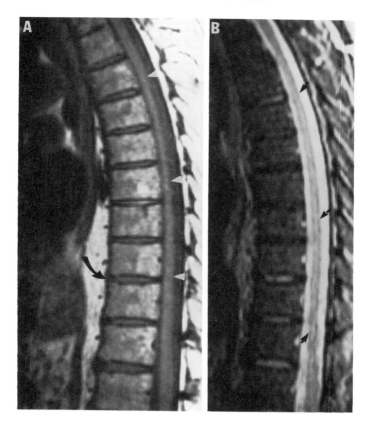

FIGURE 4. **Normal thoracic spine anatomy**—MRI. On the sagittal T1-weighted image
(A), there is excellent anatomic delineation of the vertebral bodies, intervertebral discs
(curved black arrow), and spinal cord (white arrowheads). On the sagittal cardiac gated
T2-weighted image *(B)*, as a result of the myelographic effect there is an excellent CSF-
extradural interface along with delineation of the thoracic spinal cord (black arrows).

adequately evaluated using only sagittal sequences.[132] In addition to the routine
sequences, a coronal T1-weighted sequence is helpful in the evaluation of the
spinal cord, extradural or paraspinal masses, scoliosis, and congenital anomalies.
In some centers working predominantly with tumor patients, the initial screening
study may also include an inversion recovery sequence, which provides excellent
delineation of abnormal vertebral body marrow.[30]

Lumbar Spine Protocols

Compared to the cervical and thoracic spine, the anatomical differences in
the lumbar spine that directly affect the quality of MR images include: (1) larger
size of osseous, ligamentous, and cartilaginous components; (2) increased
volume of the thecal sac; and (3) increased epidural fat. To optimally evaluate
the lumbar spine, a sagittal T1- and multiecho T2-weighted sequence and an
axial T1-weighted sequence are obtained (Fig. 5). High-resolution surface coils
are standard for all lumbar exams, and the field of view on the sagittal sequences

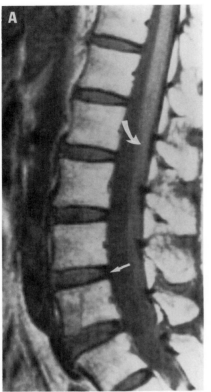

FIGURE 5. Normal lumbar spine anatomy—MRI. On the sagittal T1-weighted image *(A)*, there is excellent delineation of the vertebral bodies, intervertebral discs, thecal sac, lower thoracic cord, and conus medullaris (curved white arrow). The high signal intensity of the vertebral bodies is secondary to the fat in the cancellous marrow. There is not a well-defined interface between the posterior outer annular fibers (straight white arrow) and the cerebrospinal fluid. On the sagittal proton-density weighted image *(B)*, increased signal intensity in the disc is identified along with increased signal intensity of the cerebrospinal fluid. This results in improved delineation of the posterior annular-posterior longitudinal ligament complex (arrow). On the sagittal T2-weighted image *(C)*, increased signal intensity in the disc is identified along with a linear horizontal area of decreased signal intensity in the center of the disc representing the intranuclear cleft (arrows). There is increased signal intensity in the cerebrospinal fluid creating a myelographic effect and providing an excellent CSF-extradural interface. *(Figure continued)*.

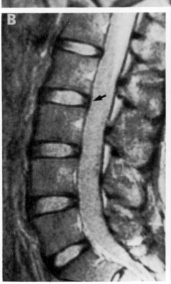

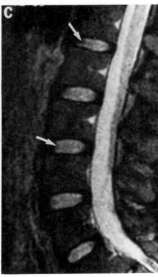

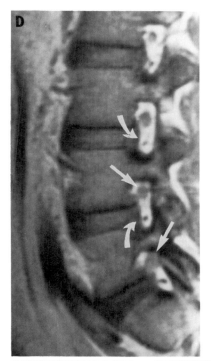

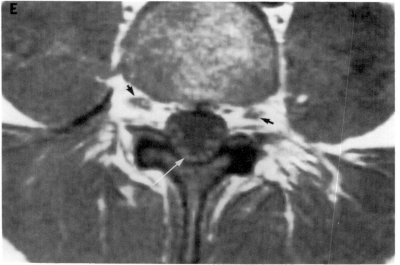

FIGURE 5 *(continued)*. On the sagittal T1-weighted image *(D)* through the intervertebral canals, there is excellent delineation of the dorsal root ganglia (straight white arrows) positioned subjacent to the vertebral pedicles. The posterolateral margin of the discs (curved white arrows) is well delineated. On the axial T1-weighted image *(E)*, there is excellent delineation of the individual nerve roots (long white arrow) in the thecal sac. The presence of fat in the epidural space and intervertebral canals provides an excellent soft tissue interface to evaluate nerve roots (short black arrows), ligaments, and osseous elements.

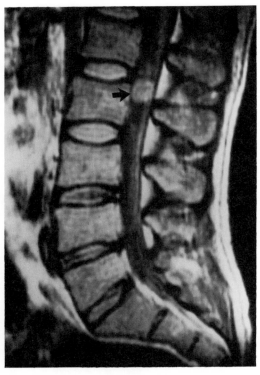

FIGURE 6. **Ependymoma of the conus medullaris**—MRI. On the evaluation of a patient presenting with low back pain, the sagittal proton-density weighted image demonstrated an unsuspected ependymoma (arrow) of the conus medullaris.

should include the region from the thoracolumbar junction, including the conus medullaris, to the sacrum (Fig. 6). Sagittal T1-weighted images are optimal in the evaluation of spinal anatomy, medullary bone, discovertebral joints, intervertebral canals, facet joints, thecal sac, conus medullaris, and extradural space. Axial T1-weighted images provide excellent delineation of the thecal sac, extradural space, facet joints, ligamenta flava, nerve roots, intervertebral canals, and paraspinal soft tissue. The importance of a sagittal T2-weighted sequence resides in the assessment of disc degeneration and herniation, marrow edema, abnormal fluid accumulations, extradural masses, and intrathecal disease. A sagittal proton-density sequence (long TR/short TE) is helpful in the evaluation of the posterior annular-posterior ligamentous complex, ligamenta flava, the central and intervertebral canals, facet joints, and posterior elements,[64] and can be obtained as part of a multiecho sagittal sequence. Slice thickness on sagittal sequences is 4–5 mm with an interslice gap of 1 mm, and on axial sequences slice thickness is 4–5 mm with an interslice gap of 1–2 mm. Contiguous axial images are obtained from the L2–3 or L3–4 disc level to the L5–S1 disc level.

CLINICAL APPLICATIONS

The purpose of an imaging study is to delineate and characterize normal and abnormal tissue. To maximize information obtained from any imaging study of the spine, it is first necessary to thoroughly understand normal spinal anatomy and the natural history of spinal diseases.[70,137] Diagnostic examinations provide information about dynamic disease processes manifesting a spectrum of disorders.

The transformation of diagnostic data into useful clinical information is directly dependent upon the level of expertise of the clinician interpreting the study.

Degenerative Spinal Disease

When describing the pathomorphologic changes in degenerative spinal disease, it is helpful to consider each disc level as a three-joint complex or motion segment with the intervertebral disc and facet joints biomechanically linked to form a functional spinal unit.[87] This will promote the critical evaluation of the entire MRI or CT/MPR study and not simply focus on one component, e.g., disc herniation, when evaluating a patient presenting with pain or neural dysfunction.

Disc Degeneration. Both MRI and CT/MPR provide excellent delineation of morphologic changes in disc herniation (Fig. 7). The major difference between the imaging modalities resides in the ability of MRI to delineate pathoanatomic and chemical changes of a degenerating disc prior to morphologic abnormalities of disc contour. Both the nucleus pulposus and annulus fibrosus consist mainly of water, collagen, and proteoglycans, with the major differences being the relative concentration of the components, level of hydration, and the particular type of collagen that predominates.[57] On T2-weighted images, the high signal intensity in the central portion of the disc originates from both the nucleus pulposus and inner annular fibers.[184] The signal intensity in the disc is related to its state of hydration and the physiochemical state of discal tissue.[58,77] On T2-weighted images, the outer annular fibers demonstrate very low signal intensity, as does the adjacent posterior longitudinal ligament.[128] With aging, there is a gradual breakdown of proteoglycans in the nucleus, gradual desiccation of the mucoid nuclear material, and loss of anatomic delineation between the nucleus and inner annular fibers.[109] Over the age of 30, an intranuclear cleft is identified in normal discs on T2-weighted MR images, and this represents normal ingrowth of fibrous tissue.[1]

Both experimentally and clinically, it appears that the development of a radial annular tear may be the necessary step in the development of disc degeneration or herniation.[99,185] It is now possible with MRI to delineate small tears in the outer annulus on T2-weighted[185] (Fig. 8) and gadolinium-DTPA (Gd-DTPA) enhanced T1-weighted images.[143] When the radial tear communicates with the nucleus, the disc will begin to degenerate and demonstrate decreased signal intensity on T2-weighted images. With communicating radial tears, displacement of the nuclear material is possible with resultant disc herniation. Displacement of the nuclear material into the region of the outer annular-posterior longitudinal ligament complex will cause altered morphology of the periphery of the disc, resulting in a focal protrusion of the disc beyond the margin of the vertebral endplates. Both MRI and CT/MPR provide excellent delineation of these contour changes.[84,178] As long as the disc material is contained by the outer annular fibers or the posterior longitudinal ligament, the herniation is designated a contained herniation.

With the superb soft-tissue resolution of MR imaging, it is possible to determine whether the disc material is contained by the outer annular-ligamentous complex or has extruded through this complex, becoming an extruded, noncontained, disc herniation[62] (Fig. 9). This information is important given the implementation of percutaneous discectomy[110] and performance of chemonucleolysis. It is also important as an indicator of surgical outcome for lumbar disc herniation.[81] The diagnosis of disc extrusion on CT studies is dependent on the

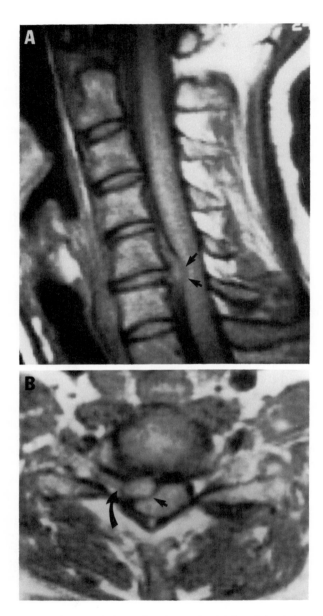

FIGURE 7. **C5–6 disc herniation.** On the sagittal T1-weighted image of the MRI examination *(A)*, there is a large posterior disc herniation (arrows) compressing the spinal cord. The axial T1-weighted image *(B)* is needed to assess the configuration of the herniation, degree of cord compression (short black arrow), and obstruction of the entrance zone of the right intervertebral canal (curved black arrow). *(Figure continued.)*

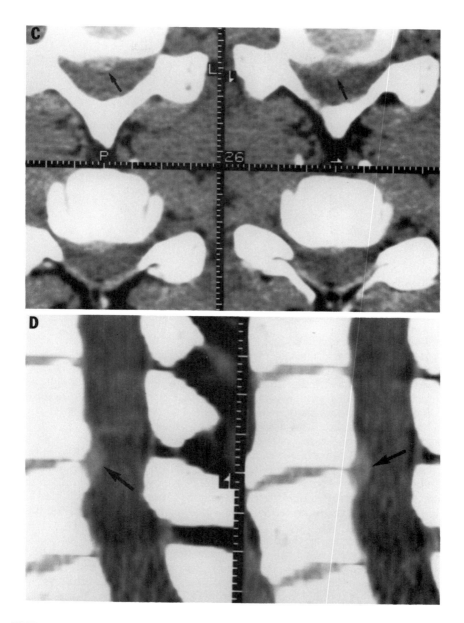

FIGURE 7 *(continued).* On the CT/MPR examination of another patient, axial *(C)* and sagittal *(D)* images demonstrate a posterior disc herniation (black arrows) at the C5–6 disc level. The morphology of the disc herniation is well delineated, but it is not possible to determine the degree of spinal cord compression.

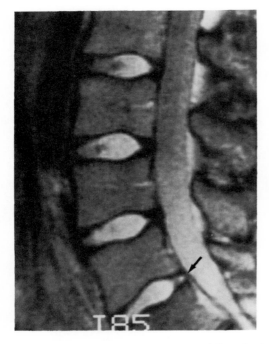

FIGURE 8. Posterior annular fissure—MRI. On the sagittal T2-weighted image at the L5–S1 level, there is a posterior annular fissure (arrow) demonstrating increased signal intensity.

configuration of the herniated disc.[50,59] Axial images obtained on either MRI or CT/MPR studies are needed to evaluate neural displacement or impingement and posterolateral or lateral disc herniations.

After disc material has penetrated through the posterior longitudinal ligament, it is possible for a portion of the disc material to separate from the disc of origin and become a sequestered fragment. In one prospective MRI study, 80% of sequestered disc fragments demonstrated hyperintensity on T2-weighted images compared to the degenerated disc of origin, whereas the remaining 20% were isointense.[106] In the same study, the accuracy of MRI in differentiating sequestered disc fragments from other forms of lumbar disc herniation was 85% compared to a 65% accuracy for CT-myelography. The differential diagnosis of a sequestered disc fragment includes epidural abscess,[132] extradural tumor,[163] conjoined nerve root,[130] nerve root sheath tumor or cyst,[61] and epidural hematoma.[98]

Following herniation, the disc will continue to degenerate and on an MRI study the degenerated disc will demonstrate decreased signal intensity. Disc herniations associated with normal signal intensity from the disc have been reported, and one study demonstrated normal signal intensity in discs that were abnormal morphologically on discography.[187] To date, there have been no prospective studies to determine the length of time necessary for a normally hydrated disc to become desiccated after it herniates. Occasionally there may be fluid containing fissures in a degenerated disc, along with ingrowth of granulation tissue,[33] which demonstrates increased signal intensity on T2-weighted images. This should not be confused with an inflammatory process.[113] Calcification or gas in the disc may be difficult to detect on T2-weighted images due to the decreased signal intensity in the severely degenerated disc and lack of MR signal

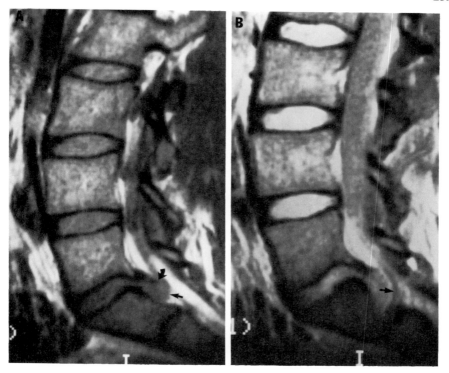

FIGURE 9.   L5–S1 disc extrusion—MRI. On the sagittal proton-density weighted image *(A)* at the L5–S1 disc level, there is a posterior disc extrusion (straight arrow) that has penetrated through the posterior annular-posterior longitudinal ligament complex (curved arrow). On the T2-weighted image *(B)*, the posterior displacement of the right S1 nerve root (arrow) by the disc extrusion is demonstrated.

from the calcium or gas. T1-weighted or gradient echo images are more useful in delineating a vacuum phenomenon or disc calcification.[117]

In addition to depicting the degenerative changes of a disc, MRI is sensitive to degenerative changes in the adjacent vertebral body endplates. Modic[120] has demonstrated pathologic alterations of the vertebral body marrow adjacent to discs undergoing degeneration. With type I endplate degeneration, there is a decreased signal intensity in the subchondral cancellous bone on a T1-weighted image and increased signal intensity on a T2-weighted image (Fig. 10). The region of altered signal intensity pathologically represents prominent fibrovascular tissue in the marrow adjacent to the vertebral body endplate. Compared to normal marrow, type II endplate degenerative changes, which pathologically represent increased fat in the subchondral bone marrow, demonstrate hyperintensity on T1-weighted images and slight hyperintensity or isointensity on T2-weighted images. Type III endplate degenerative changes represent coarsening and thickening of the subchondral trabeculae, which is depicted on T1- and T2-weighted images as decreased signal intensity. On a CT/MPR evaluation, only endplate sclerosis can be delineated, and this is not necessarily correlated to type III changes identified by MRI.

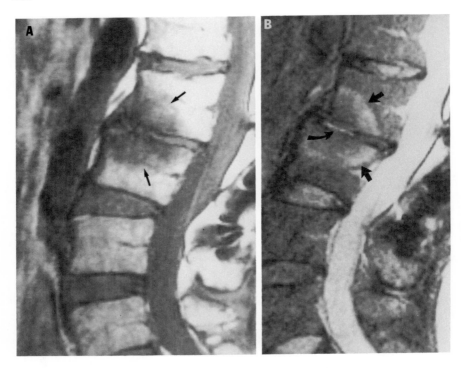

FIGURE 10. **Type I endplate degenerative changes**—MRI. On the sagittal T1-weighted image *(A)* at the L2–3 disc level, moderately severe decreased disc height is present along with a minimal retrolisthesis. There is a hemispheric region of decreased signal intensity (straight black arrows) in the cancellous bone adjacent to the degenerative discovertebral joint. On the T2-weighted image *(B)*, there is increased signal intensity (straight black arrows) in the cancellous bone. Increased signal intensity is present in the anterior portion of the disc space (curved black arrow), most likely representing fluid in degenerative fissures.

With the excellent characterization of normal and abnormal discs by MRI, it is now possible to noninvasively study the natural history of disc degeneration and herniation. The sensitivity of MRI to early changes of disc degeneration should help in the evaluation of patients with intervertebral disc resorption[82] or internal disc disruption.[11] Multiple studies have been reported describing the excellent sensitivity, specificity, and accuracy of MRI[39,48] and CT[34,47,50,71,112] in the diagnosis of discal disease. Even though a disc herniation is identified, it is important to realize the relatively common occurrence of asymptomatic disc herniations in the cervical,[167] thoracic,[180] and lumbar spine.[133,176,177] With increased utilization of MRI, it has also become clear that disc degeneration and herniation afflict the adolescent age population[45,46] as well as young adults,[125] in addition to patients over the age of 30.

Facet Arthrosis. As part of a three-joint complex, the facet joints are biomechanically linked to the discovertebral joint. Altered functional status of one component of the complex may induce degeneration of another component of the spinal unit. The size and orientation of the facet joints differ at different levels of the spine and, representing diarthrodial joints, are subject to painful degeneration.[12,121] In the evaluation of facet orientation,[66,86,171] and facet arthrosis, CT is unsurpassed.[27] Early erosions, cystic changes, hyperostosis, and facet capsular calcification are clearly delineated on a CT examination. Degenerative changes of the facet joints resolved by MRI include facet hypertrophy, osteophytic spurring, cartilage narrowing, joint effusions, and capsular hypertrophy[64] (Fig. 11). Cartilage thickness is difficult to measure accurately because of partial volume averaging and chemical shift artifacts. Gradient echo sequences may prove useful in the evaluation of facet degenerative changes, particularly when evaluating articular cartilage.

Spinal Stenosis. Spinal stenosis is defined as local, segmental, or generalized narrowing of the central or intervertebral canals by bony or soft tissue elements that may lead to encroachment on the neural structures. The narrowing may involve the bony canal alone or the dural sac, or both.[4] The degenerative changes most often associated with stenosis include hyperostotic spurring of the vertebral body endplates, uncinate processes, and facet joints, along with hypertrophy of the ligamenta flava and anterior facet capsules.[79,101,137] The initial size of the central and intervertebral canals is an important factor in determining whether degenerative changes will cause neural impingement or compression. The goal of MRI and CT/MPR in the evaluation of the patient presenting with radiculopathy, myeloradiculopathy, or myelopathy is not just to demonstrate that stenosis is present, but to define the relative contributions of each component of the stenotic process.

In the evaluation of patients presenting with cervical myelopathy or radiculopathy, thin-section high-resolution CT has been an excellent screening exam of the cervical spine.[112] CT does not directly demonstrate neural impingement or compression and frequently a contrast study is still needed preoperatively.[34] In the evaluation of cervical spondylosis, CT/MPR is excellent in differentiating between disc herniations and spondylotic spurs (Fig. 12). This is more difficult with MRI because of thicker sections[21] and variable signal intensity in degenerative osseous ridges.[115] The strength of MRI is in its clear delineation of the effect of the spondylotic changes on the neural elements in the central and intervertebral canals (Fig. 13). In several recent series, excellent results with MRI compared to CT-myelography and myelography have been demonstrated when evaluating patients with radiculopathy and myelopathy.[21,115] In addition to the routine sagittal and axial MRI sequences, gradient echo sequences are beneficial in defining the exact etiology of stenosis.[72,103] In the cervical spine, there is a strong association pathologically between degenerative changes of the discovertebral joint and uncinate spurs at the same motion segment. Many patients presenting with myelopathy secondary to spondylotic changes will also have an associated radiculopathy.[36] CT/MPR, with its thin sections, is optimal in the evaluation of uncinate spurs projecting into the intervertebral canals. Oblique imaging of the intervertebral canals adds information to a standard MRI exam and is included if the intervertebral canals cannot be adequately evaluated on standard sequences.[118]

In the evaluation of patients with myelopathy or myeloradiculopathy, it is important to accurately determine the size of the central spinal canal.[44] A true osseous diameter can only be obtained from axial images orthogonal to the long axis of the cervical central canal or by sagittal images.[159] CT/MPR, with its excellent osseous delineation, currently provides the most accurate osseous measurements. Osseous stenosis does not necessarily cause cervical myelopathy, and the great advantage of MRI over CT when evaluating stenosis is its

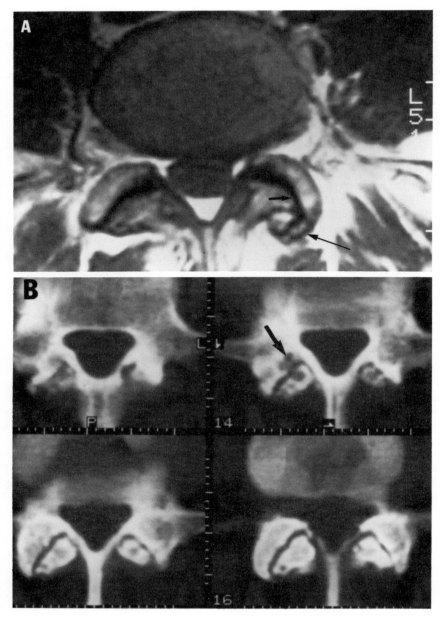

FIGURE 11. Lumbar facet arthrosis. On the axial proton-density weighted image of the MRI examination *(A)*, degeneration of the left facet joint is identified with narrowing of the articular cartilage (short arrow) and osteophytic spurring of the dorsal surface (long arrow) of the left superior articular process. On the CT/MPR evaluation of the lumbar spine *(B)*, there is excellent delineation of subchondral cystic changes (black arrow) involving the facet joints.

demonstration of what effect the degenerative processes and/or a developmentally narrowed central canal have on the neural structures. Patients presenting with myelopathic symptoms frequently have degenerative spondylotic changes superimposed on a developmentally narrowed central canal.[41] In recent studies, the best predictor of the clinical course in myelopathic patients, the effect of surgical intervention, and the pathologic changes of the spinal cord is the degree of cord compression and measurement of cord volume.[53,54] A recent MRI study evaluated 668 patients with chronic cervical cord compression and demonstrated high signal intensity within the spinal cord on T2-weighted or proton-density images in 14.8% of the patients. This finding was directly related to increased spinal cord compression and to the severity of clinical myelopathy. Patients with high signal intensity areas responded less favorably to surgical or medical treatment.[165] An exciting future application of MRI is the dynamic evaluation of the cervical spine in flexion and extension.[31] MRI is also excellent in the delineation of pathologic processes that may mimic spondylotic cervical myelopathy, including spinal cord tumors, intra- and extradural masses, metastatic disease, and demyelinating processes.

In the lumbar spine, it has become clear that patients of any age may present with disc degeneration superimposed on a stenotic process or may present with isolated stenosis as a cause of leg or back pain.[24,69] The classification of spinal stenosis as congenital, developmental, and acquired is extremely helpful when evaluating a small spinal canal.[173,174] **Congenital stenosis** is due to disturbed fetal development and may occur as one element of a congenital malformation of the lumbar spine. **Developmental stenosis** is a growth disturbance of the posterior elements, involving the pedicles, lamina, and articular processes, resulting in decreased volume of the spinal canal.[139] A true midline osseous sagittal diameter measuring less than 12 mm is considered relative stenosis, and a diameter of less than 10 mm, absolute stenosis. This diameter is measured from the middle of the posterior surface of the vertebral body to the point of junction of the base of the spinous process and laminae. With relative stenosis, the reserve capacity of the spinal canal is reduced and a small disc herniation or early degenerative changes may cause symptomatic stenosis in both the young and the older population. **Acquired stenosis** is the narrowing of the central or intervertebral canals by degenerative changes of the discovertebral joints, facet joints, and ligamenta flava[151,152,173] (Fig. 14). In a prospective study, 60 patients with suspected lumbar disc herniations and/or central stenosis were studied with surface coil MRI, CT, and/or myelography, and the results were compared to the findings at surgery. Surgical findings of stenosis agreed with the MRI findings in 77%, CT findings in 79%, and myelographic findings in 54%.[114] This study did not differentiate between central and intervertebral canal stenosis, and the study also did not include multiplanar reformations, which are helpful in the CT evaluation of central and intervertebral canal stenosis.[93,107] In recent reports, the cross-sectional area of the thecal sac correlated best to stenotic symptoms.[14] MRI is ideally suited to evaluate the true sagittal dimension and cross-sectional area of the thecal sac, thus obviating the need for CT-myelography.

The importance of intervertebral canal stenosis as a cause of radicular symptoms[131] has been well documented, along with its significance in failed back surgery.[24] Considering that all intervertebral canals in the spinal column have a vertical and horizontal dimension, as well as a length (5 mm in the cervical to 12 mm in the lumbar), the canals are truly a three-dimensional structure and

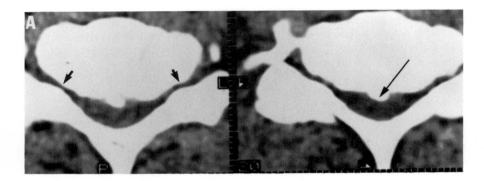

FIGURE 12. Severe stenosis of the cervical central and intervertebral canals—CT/ MPR. On the axial images (*A* [*above*] and *B* [*opposite page*]), severe central (long arrow) and intervertebral canal (short arrows) stenosis is well delineated. The sagittal reconstructed images (*C* [*opposite page*] and *D* [*below*]) are optimal to evaluate the central spondylotic ridges (straight arrows) and the uncinate spurs (curved arrows).

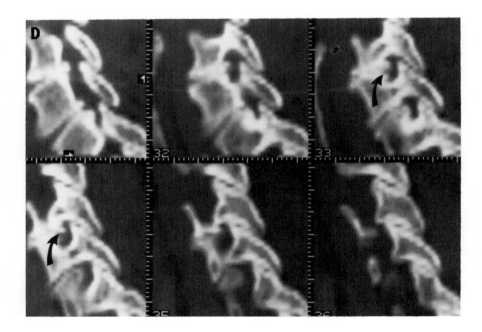

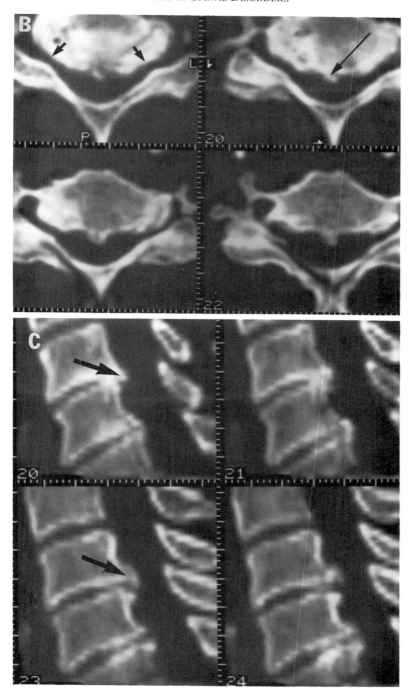

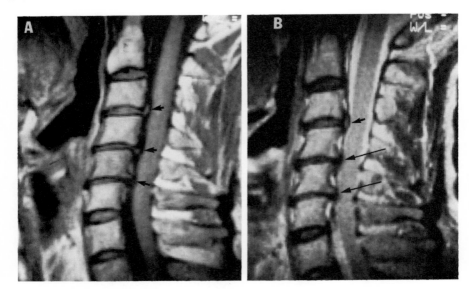

FIGURE 13. **Multilevel cervical spondylosis superimposed on developmental stenosis—**
MRI. On the sagittal T1-weighted image *(A),* degenerative changes are identified at the
C3–4, C4–5, and C5–6 disc levels (arrows). The extradural space is poorly defined due to
the isointensity of the cerebrospinal fluid, posterior annular-posterior longitudinal
ligament complex, and vertebral body cortex. On the sagittal cardiac gated T2-weighted
image *(B),* with the increased signal intensity in the cerebrospinal fluid, a posterior disc
herniation at the C3–4 disc level causing minimal cord impingement (short arrow) is now
easily identified. Changes of cervical spondylosis are present at the C4–5 and C5–6 disc
levels with spondylotic ridges (long arrows) causing mild cord impingement. There is
decreased AP diameter of the central spinal canal from the C3–4 level on a developmental
basis, with resultant decreased functional spinal canal volume predisposing to cord
impingement.

should not be designated as foramen. Pathologic changes of any component of
the intervertebral canal may impinge or compress a nerve root. The intervertebral
canal at the L5–S1 disc level is unique in its morphometry, and due to its length
it may be stenotic at its entrance, middle, or exit zone. The most common
etiology of stenosis at this level is osteophytic spurs projecting off the inferior
endplate of L5 and less commonly the superior endplate of S1[13,137] (Fig. 15).
Extracanalicular ("far out") stenosis[181] may also occur at the L5–S1 disc level in
patients with spondylolisthesis or elderly patients with scoliosis and disc
degeneration.[65] This stenosis is secondary to apposition of the base of the
transverse process of L5 to the adjacent sacral ala. In addition, osseous spurs may
project off the lateral margin of the vertebral body endplates of L5 and S1 and
impinge the L5 nerve root in the paravertebral gutter. The pathoanatomy of this
region is excellently demonstrated by CT/MPR and by three-dimensional images
created from the CT data (Fig. 16).

Degenerative spondylolisthesis is an important cause of central canal
stenosis (Fig. 17) and most frequently involves the L4–5 disc level.[100] Disc
degeneration along with degenerative changes of sagittally oriented facet joints[149]
predispose the motion segment to an anterolisthesis that rarely progresses

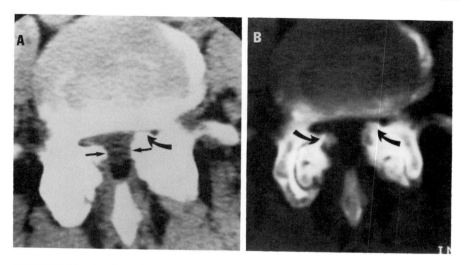

FIGURE 14. Moderately severe central canal stenosis at the L4–5 disc level—CT. On the axial images (*A* and *B*), severe facet degenerative changes are delineated with hyperostotic spurs projecting off the anteromedial margin of the facet joints (curved black arrows), causing stenosis of the subarticular lateral recesses. The osseous spurring and hypertrophy of the facet joints are causing moderate compression of the thecal sac (straight black arrows).

beyond a grade I slip due to the intact neural arch. Hyperostotic spurs projecting off the anteromedial margin of the facet joints, hypertrophy of the ligamenta flava, annular redundancy, and an anterolisthesis can result in severe central canal and subarticular lateral recess stenosis. There is usually at least mild narrowing of the intervertebral canals in the cephalocaudal direction secondary to the decreased disc height and the anterolisthesis.

Isthmic spondylolysis represents a fracture of the pars interarticularis, but since the presenting symptoms of adolescent and adult patients with spondylolysis are usually related to secondary degenerative changes, it has been included in this section. Fragmentation and hypertrophy of the pars interarticularis can lead to a narrowed central spinal canal. Stenosis of the intervertebral canals is frequently identified and may be secondary to the anterolisthesis, the hypertrophied pars interarticularis, degenerative spurs projecting off the vertebral body endplates, and disc or soft tissue encroachment.[40,182] Spondylolysis associated with spondylolisthesis at the L5–S1 disc level frequently results in stenosis of the intervertebral canals in a cephalocaudal direction.[75] CT/MPR is optimal in the depiction of fragmentation of hypertrophy of the pars interarticularis and in the evaluation of osseous degenerative changes.[145] MRI is excellent in the evaluation of neural impingement or disc degeneration, which is more prevalent in patients with spondylolysis at both the level of the spondylolytic defects[164] and at the superjacent disc level[63,145] (Fig. 18).

Spinal Trauma

The optimal treatment of cervical cord injury secondary to vertebral fracture and/or dislocation is still in the process of evolution.[35] MRI provides the first

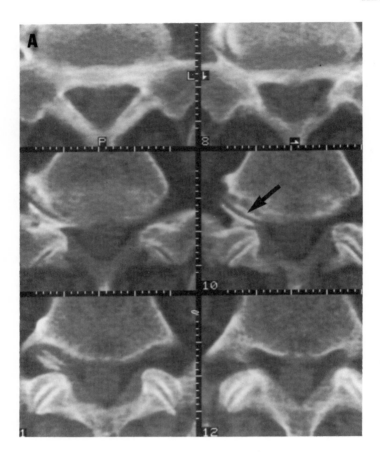

FIGURE 15. **Intervertebral canal stenosis at the L5–S1 disc level**—CT/MPR. On the axial image *(A)*, the spondylotic spurs (straight arrow) are identified, projecting into the right intervertebral canal. *(Figure continued.)*

noninvasive imaging procedure to directly assess the degree of dural and spinal cord compression and pathologic spinal cord changes.[6,92] Injury to posterior ligaments, osseous structures, soft tissues, and discovertebral joints can also be evaluated on the standard MRI examination.[42,111,169] The value of MRI in diagnosing spinal cord hemorrhage, edema, and neural compression has been well documented. Recent studies have demonstrated that neurologic recovery was insignificant in patients with intramedullary spinal cord hemorrhage or extensive contusion, but recovery in neurologic function was observed with patients demonstrating only cord edema.[92,150] The sagittal T1-weighted sequence demonstrated altered spinal cord morphology, but the sagittal T2-weighted sequence was the most important for delineating abnormal signal intensity from hemorrhage, contusion, or edema in the spinal cord. The evaluation of the cervico-occipital junction and C1–2 relationship in patients with an atlantoaxial subluxation[89] can now be easily assessed with MRI.[22] In one study comparing MRI to CT-myelography in the evaluation of cervical trauma, MRI was superior

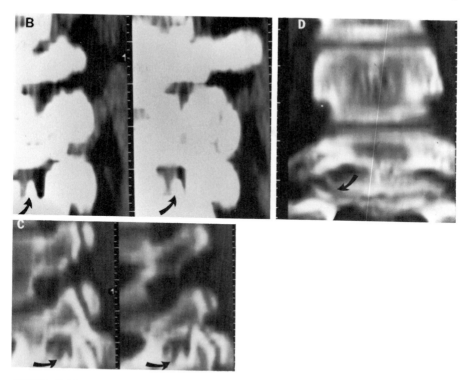

FIGURE 15 *(continued).* The sagittal (*B* and *C*) and coronal *(D)* reconstructed images optimally delineate the degree of stenosis secondary to the degenerative spurs (curved arrows).

except in the delineation of cervical spine fractures.[111] Fractures or malalignment of the posterior elements is optimally evaluated utilizing a CT/MPR examination[8] (Fig. 19). In the evaluation of a chronically injured spinal cord, MRI is the optimal study to differentiate myelomalacia from post-traumatic cysts.[134]

The role of MRI and computed tomography is complementary in the evaluation of spinal trauma involving the thoracolumbar junction and lumbosacral spine. CT/MPR provides excellent delineation of fractures and deformation of the vertebral bodies or posterior elements,[18,19,55,68,108,124] whereas MRI is optimal in evaluating the thecal sac an conus medullaris (Fig. 20). In one study, neurologic morbidity was related to the level of the conus medullaris and patency of the ventral subarachnoid space demonstrated on the MRI examination.[10]

Spinal Tumors

Patients with tumors involving the central spinal cord or vertebrae may present with a rapidly progressive myeloradiculopathy, but most frequently their symptomatology is subacute or chronic in nature. In the evaluation of spinal tumors, it is helpful to classify tumor location as: (1) intramedullary, (2) intradural-extramedullary, (3) extradural, and (4) osseous. Some tumors may be found in two locations, particularly in the case of metastatic disease that involves the vertebral body and extradural space.

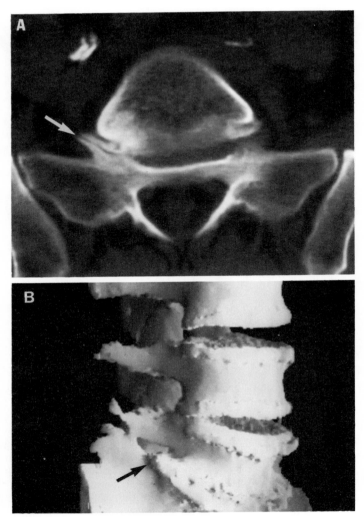

FIGURE 16.   **Exit zone stenosis of the right intervertebral canal at the L5–S1 disc level—**
CT. On the axial CT image *(A)*, spondylotic spurs (arrow) are identified projecting into
the exit zone of the right intervertebral canal and lateral to the vertebral body endplates.
The size and the position of the spondylotic ridges (arrow) are easier to appreciate on the
three-dimensional image *(B)* created from the CT data.

MRI has rapidly become the imaging study of choice in the assessment of
intramedullary lesions of the spinal cord.[95,162] In addition to delineating morphologic alterations of the spinal cord, MRI is able to characterize the nature of the
intramedullary disease due to the difference in signal intensity of blood, tumor,
and cyst compared to the normal spinal cord. The intravenous administration of
gadolinium-DTPA is extremely helpful in the delineation of spinal cord tumors[161]
(Fig. 21) and in the differentiation of a benign from a malignant syrinx.[162,179] In

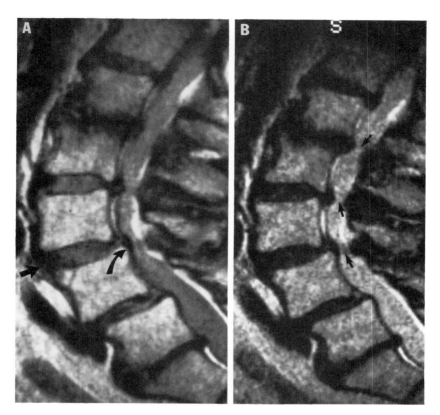

FIGURE 17. **Multilevel degenerative changes of the lumbar spine**—MRI. On the sagittal proton-density weighted image *(A)*, multilevel degenerative changes are identified. A degenerative anterolisthesis is present at the L3–4 disc level (short straight arrow), causing moderately severe central canal stenosis (curved black arrow). On the sagittal T2-weighted image *(B)*, disc degeneration and decreased signal intensity are identified at all disc levels. Increased signal intensity of the cerebrospinal fluid facilitates the evaluation of the degree of multilevel central canal stenosis (arrows).

addition to primary and metastatic malignant tumors in the spinal cord,[49] enhancement with gadolinium-DTPA has also been reported with spinal cord infarcts, myelomalacia, myelitis, multiple sclerosis,[104] sarcoidosis,[122] and arterio-venous malformations.[37]

In the evaluation of intradural-extramedullary tumors, the intravenous injection of Gd-DTPA transforms a relatively insensitive standard MRI examination into an extremely effective exam for depicting leptomeningeal spread of tumor.[91] Compared to myelography and CT-myelography, recent studies have demonstrated MRI to be more sensitive and specific in the delineation of extradural masses causing cord compression.[26] CT/MPR continues to be optimal for demonstrating involvement of the posterior elements or vertebral cortex by primary or metastatic tumors.

For evaluating spinal dysraphism, MRI has quickly become the initial screening examination to assess spinal cord morphology, positions of the conus

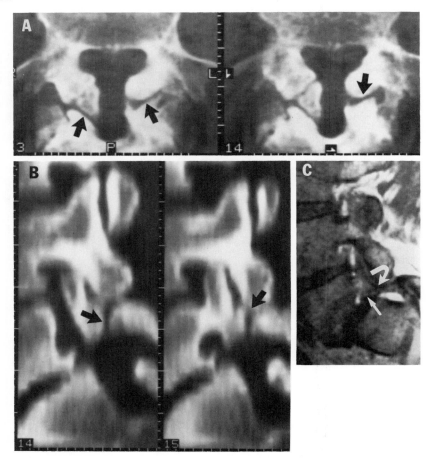

FIGURE 18.   Isthmic spondylolysis. On the CT/MPR examination, axial *(A)* and sagittal *(B)* images demonstrate spondylolytic defects (arrows) involving the L5 pars interarticularis. On the sagittal T1-weighted image of the MRI examination *(C)*, the spondylolytic defect (curved arrow) involving the L5 pars interarticularis is difficult to delineate. There is excellent delineation of the cephalocaudal narrowing of the intervertebral canal and compression of the L5 nerve root (straight arrow).

medullaris and filum terminale, and to identify associated lipomatous traction lesions.[5,135]

Vertebral Body Marrow Disorders

MRI is extremely sensitive to any pathologic process that replaces the normal fat in the bone marrow. T1- and T2-weighted sequences are needed to characterize the pathologic alterations.[175] In addition to the standard T1- and T-2 weighted sequences, inversion recovery, gradient echo,[153] and chemical shift imaging[140] are also employed in the workup of marrow disorders. MRI is extremely sensitive to alterations in the vertebral body marrow but lacks specificity as to the etiology of the various pathologic processes involving the vertebrae.[160] Any disorder or therapeutic procedure resulting in loss of myeloid

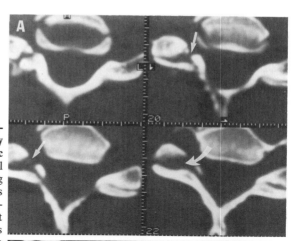

FIGURE 19. **Posterior ele-**
ment fracture and partial rotary
subluxation at the C5–6 disc
level—CT/MPR. On the axial
images *(A)*, a fracture involving
the base of the right lateral mass
of C6 (straight arrows) is identified and diastasis of the right
facet joint (curved arrow). It is
extremely difficult to evaluate
the degree of malalignment
using only axial images. On the
sagittal images *(B)*, the anterior
subluxation of the inferior articular process of C5 (straight
white arrows) is delineated along
with the impacted fracture of
the C6 lateral mass (black
arrows). The diastasis of the
C5–6 facet joint (curved white
arrow) is also well delineated.
The coronal images *(C)* are optimal to delineate the orientation
of the fracture (arrows) involving the base of the lateral mass
of C6.

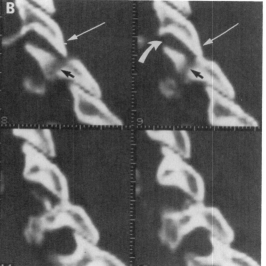

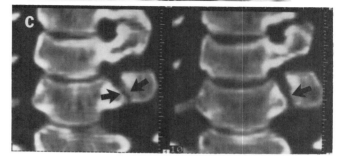

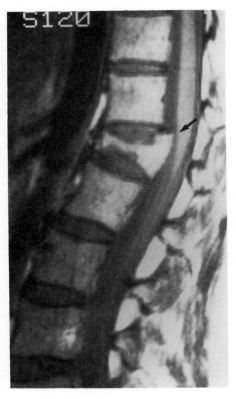

FIGURE 20. Benign compression fracture of the L1 vertebral body—MRI. On the sagittal T1-weighted image, there is a benign compression fracture of the L1 vertebral body. The retropulsion of the vertebral body results in minimal impingement of the conus medullaris (arrow). Diffuse decreased signal intensity in the cancellous bone of the L3, L4, and L5 vertebral bodies is identified and represents metastatic disease.

elements, e.g., aplastic anemia[158] or radiation therapy,[136] will also demonstrate altered signal intensity in the marrow on an MRI examination.

Spinal Infection

In an adult, infection involving the spinal column usually affects the vertebral bodies and intervening disc. MRI should be the initial screening study in the evaluation of vertebral osteomyelitis. The MRI findings on sagittal images include: (1) confluent decreased signal intensity in the vertebral bodies and intervertebral disc, with inability to discern a margin between the disc and the adjacent vertebral bodies on a T1-weighted image; (2) increased signal intensity in the vertebral bodies adjacent to the intervertebral disc on a T2-weighted image; and (3) abnormal configuration and increased signal intensity of the intervertebral disc and absence of the intranuclear cleft on a T2-weighted image (TR 2000–3000 ms, TE 120 ms) (Fig. 22). MRI has a reported sensitivity of 96%, specificity of 93%, and accuracy of 94% in diagnosing osteomyelitis, equaling the results of a combined bone scan and gallium study.[113] The main advantages of MRI over radionuclide studies include acquisition of significant information about the spinal cord, thecal sac, and paravertebral soft tissues. The MRI findings of nonpyogenic osteomyelitis may be atypical, suggesting neoplasm rather than infection.[157] Tuberculous spondylitis occasionally will present with focal involvement of the vertebral body or posterior elements and lack of involvement of the disc and vertebral body endplates.[170] MRI has also rapidly become the screening exam for the evaluation of epidural

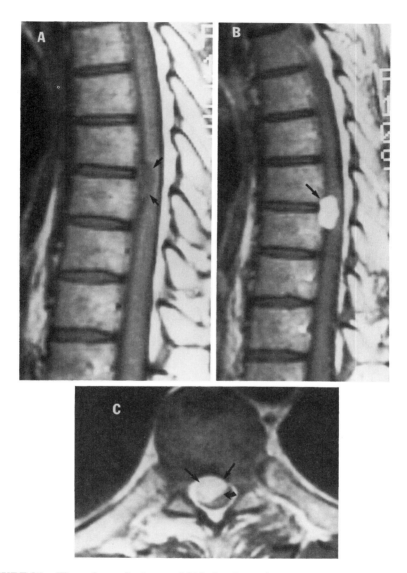

FIGURE 21.   Thoracic meningioma—MRI. On the sagittal T1-weighted image *(A)*, an anterior extradural soft tissue mass (arrows) is identified compressing the thoracic spinal cord. After the administration of gadolinium-DTPA, on the sagittal *(B)* and the axial *(C)* T1-weighted images, there is excellent delineation of the enhancing epidural mass (straight arrows). The degree of spinal cord compression (curved arrow) is best delineated on the axial image.

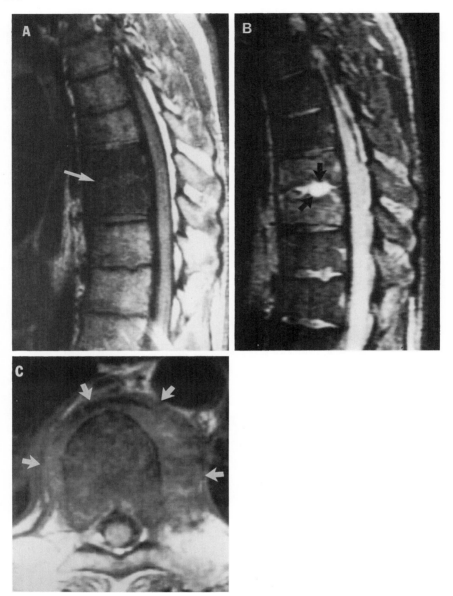

FIGURE 22. Pyogenic vertebral osteomyelitis—MRI. On the sagittal T1-weighted image *(A)*, there is a confluent area of decreased signal intensity involving the T7 and T8 vertebral bodies and the intervening disc (arrow). On the sagittal T2-weighted image *(B)*, increased signal intensity is identified in the disc space (arrows) along with diffuse increased signal intensity in the adjacent vertebral body marrow. The axial T1-weighted image *(C)* is needed to determine the degree of extension of the inflammatory process into the paravertebral soft tissue (arows).

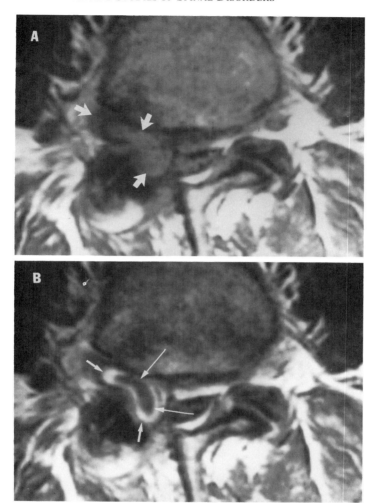

FIGURE 23. **Sequestered disc fragment**—postoperative MRI examination. On the axial T1-weighted image *(A)*, there is a large soft tissue extradural mass (arrows) interposed between the right lateral margin of the thecal sac and the right facet joint. The mass extends through the right intervertebral canal. After the administration of Gd-DTPA, on the repeat axial T1-weighted image *(B)*, a large sequestered disc fragment (long arrows) with low signal intensity is now identified surrounded by epidural fibrosis (short arrows), demonstrating high signal intensity.

abscesses.[3] In one recent study, the MRI findings were diagnostic for osteomyelitis with disc space infection associated with epidural abscesses. These findings obviated the need for CT-myelography when there was no concomitant meningitis.[132]

Postoperative Evaluation of the Spine

It is not infrequent for patients who have undergone spinal surgery to experience persistent or recurrent back pain. In one series, the most frequent

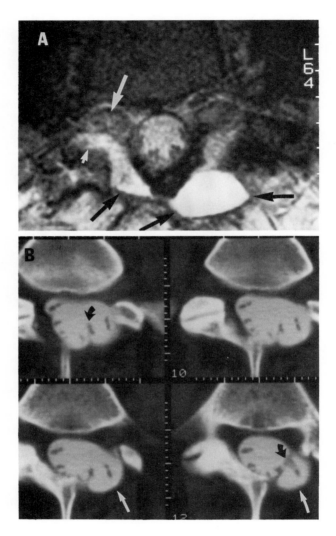

FIGURE 24.   **Postoperative pseudomeningocele.** On the MRI axial T2-weighted image *(A)*, there is a collection of fluid (black arrows) posterior to the thecal sac. The fluid extends into the right intervertebral canal (short white arrow) where it is positioned posterior to an enlarged dorsal root ganglion (large lwhite arrow). On the CT/MPR myelogram of another patient, there is excellent delineation on the axial *(B)* and coronal (*C* [*opposite page*]) images of a small pseudomeningocele (white arrows) located at the L5–S1 disc level. The displacement of the nerve roots (curved black arrows) into the pseudomeningocele is demonstrated.

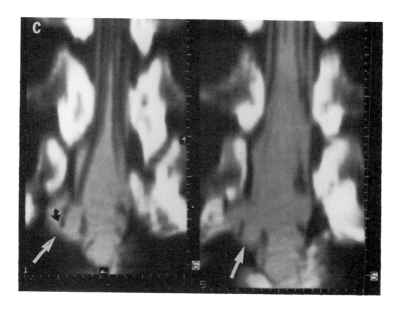

FIGURE 24. *(Continued.)*

findings to explain the patient's symptoms included stenosis of the central and intervertebral canals, disc herniation, arachnoiditis, epidural fibrosis, and direct nerve injury.[24]

MRI should be the screening evaluation if recurrent or persistent disc herniation is clinically suspected. When performing MRI examinations on the postoperative spine, the interval of time between surgery and an MRI examination is an important factor in the evaluation of MRI findings. In one recent study, there was no correlation between the immediate postoperative appearance on an MRI exam and patient symptoms, and the authors concluded that the MRI study in the immediate postoperative period was not useful to explain the etiology of persistent pain.[142] Patients with recurrent back pain or failed back surgery syndrome present with a variety of postoperative findings. Epidural fibrosis is frequently present at the operative site and typically demonstrates intermediate signal intensity on T1-weighted images and increased signal intensity on T2-weighted images.[23,78] Fibrosis is usually poorly marginated and generates no mass effect. Recurrent disc herniations typically are contiguous with the disc space, well marginated, and, compared to the disc of origin, demonstrate isointensity or hypointensity on T1-weighted images and isointensity or hyperintensity on T2-weighted images. In two studies utilizing the criteria of epidural location, morphologic configuration, signal intensity, and mass effect, MRI was extremely accurate in differentiating disc herniation from fibrosis.[23,51] The intravenous administration of Gd-DTPA has also been helpful in differentiating disc material from fibrosis[80] (Fig. 23). In the evaluation of the postoperative patient, an axial T2-weighted sequence is obtained if epidural abscess,[132] pseudomeningocele[126] (Fig. 24), or arachnoiditis[141] (Fig. 25) are clinically suspected.

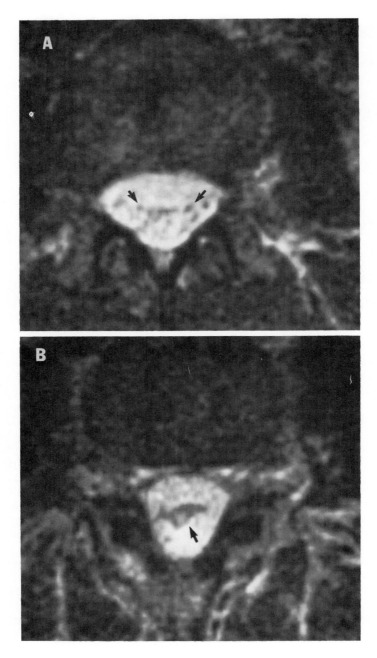

FIGURE 25. **Postoperative arachnoiditis**—MRI. On the axial T2-weighted image *(A)*, above the level of the surgical procedure, the nerve roots (arrows) have a normal appearance. At the level of surgery *(B)*, the nerve roots (arrow) are clumped in the central portion of the thecal sac.

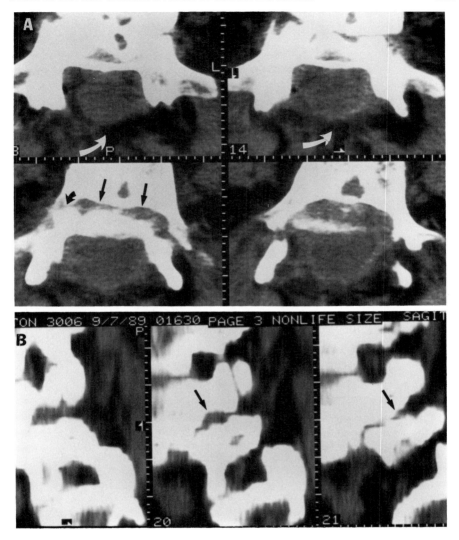

FIGURE 26. **Postoperative instability with an anterolisthesis at the L4–5 disc level**—CT/ MPR. On the axial images *(A)*, a wide posterior laminectomy (curved white arrows) is demonstrated. An anterolisthesis (straight black arrows) can be appreciated, but it is extremely difficult to determine the degree of stenosis of the intervertebral canal (curved black arrow). On the sagittal images *(B)*, severe stenosis of the L4–5 intervertebral canal (arrows) is delineated.

CT/MPR is still the screening modality of choice in the evaluation of postoperative stenosis.[20,97] With its excellent delineation of osseous structures, it is optimal when evaluating encroachment of the central or intervertebral canals secondary to a degenerative process or in the evaluation of postoperative spondylolisthesis[83,96] (Fig. 26). It is also more sensitive than MRI in the evaluation of spinal fusions[28,146] (Fig. 27) and in the delineation of postoperative fractures of the lumbar articular facets.[147]

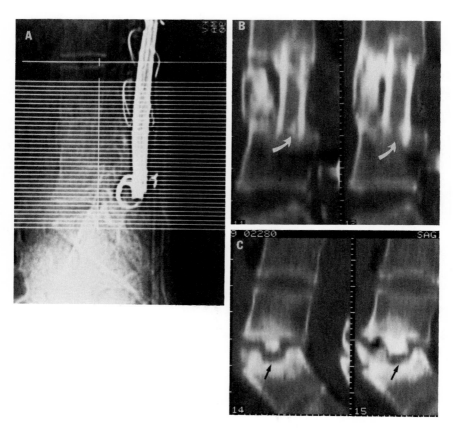

FIGURE 27. **Postoperative evaluation of interbody fusions**—CT/MPR. On the initial lateral scout view *(A)*, posterior metallic instrumentation is identified that does not preclude the excellent delineation of a solid interbody fusion (arrows) demonstrated on the sagittal *(B)* reconstructed images. On the examination of another patient, the sagittal reconstructed images *(C)* demonstrate a pseudoarthrosis of an interbody fusion (arrows) at the L5–S1 disc level.

Spondyloarthropathies

With the spine being a composite of amphiarthroses, diarthroses, and entheses, it may be affected by a variety of arthritic processes. MRI is particularly useful in evaluating patients with rheumatoid arthritis affecting the cervical spine[85] who present with symptoms of myelopathy or myeloradiculopathy. Vertical subluxation of the odontoid, atlantoaxial subluxation, or subaxial subluxation[22] are frequently identified in patients with long-standing rheumatoid arthritis. MRI can demonstrate the degree of cord impingement on both a static and dynamic examination,[38] along with abnormalities of the atlantodental interval and apophyseal joints. In patients with ankylosing spondylitis presenting with spinal pseudarthrosis[29] or fracture dislocations,[67] CT/MPR is the most sensitive study for delineating osseous deformation, but MRI is of benefit for determining whether there is neural compression.

CONCLUSION

In the evaluation of disorders of the spinal column, there are two superb diagnostic imaging modalities, CT/MPR and MRI, both of which delineate spinal pathomorphology. While the strengths of CT/MPR reside in its excellent demonstration of osseous detail and the strengths of MRI in its excellent characterization of soft tissue abnormalities, prospective controlled clinical studies are critically needed to assess the efficacy of the two imaging procedures when evaluating the myriad of disease processes that affect the spinal column. I believe it is necessary for more radiologists to become subspecialists in the evaluation of organ systems, such as the spine, if we hope to maximize the information that we obtain from these complex diagnostic modalities. With subspecialization, the radiologist can become an integral part of a multidisciplinary team of physicians caring for patients with spinal dysfunction.

REFERENCES

1. Aguila LA, Piraino DW, Modic MT, et al: The intranuclear cleft of the intervertebral disk: Magnetic resonance imaging. Radiology 155:155–158, 1985.
2. Alvarez O, Roque CT, Pampati M: Multilevel thoracic disk herniations: CT and MR studies. J Comput Assist Tomogr 12:649–652, 1988.
3. Angtuaco EJC, McConnell JR, Chadduck WM, Flanigan S: MR imaging of spinal epidural sepsis. AJR 149:1249–1253, 1987.
4. Arnoldi CC, Brodsky AE, Cauchoix J, et al: Lumbar spinal stenosis and nerve root entrapment syndromes: Definition and classification. Clin Orthop Rel Res 115:4–5, 1976.
5. Barnes PD, Lester PD, Yamanashi WS, Prince JR: MRI in infants and children with spinal dysraphism. AJR 147:339–346, 1986.
6. Beers GJ, Raque GH, Wagner GG, et al: MR imaging in acute cervical spine trauma. J Comput Assist Tomogr 12:755–761, 1988.
7. Bellon EM, Haacke EM, Coleman PE, et al: MR artifacts: A review. AJR 147:1271–1281, 1986.
8. Bergström K, Nyberg G, Pech P, Rauschning W, Ytterbergh C: Multiplanar spinal anatomy: Comparison of CT and cryomicrotomy in postmortem specimens. AJNR 4:590–592, 1983.
9. Berns DH, Blaser SI, Modic MT: Magnetic resonance imaging of the spine. Clin Orthop Rel Res 244:78–100, 1989.
10. Blumenkopf B, Juneau PA III: Magnetic resonance imaging (MRI) of thoracolumbar fractures. J Spinal Disorders 1:144–150, 1988.
11. Blumenthal SL, Baker J, Dossett A, Selby DK: The role of anterior lumbar fusion for internal disc disruption. Spine 13:566–569, 1988.
12. Bogduk N, Marsland A: The cervical zygapophyseal joints as a source of neck pain. Spine 13:610–617, 1988.
13. Bohatirchuk F: The ageing vertebral column (macro- and historadiographical study). Br J Radiol 28:389–404, 1955.
14. Bolender NF, Schonstrom NSR, Spengler DM: Role of computed tomography and myelography in the diagnosis of central spinal stenosis. J Bone Joint Surg 67A:240–245, 1985.
15. Bottomley PA: Human in vivo NMR spectroscopy in diagnostic medicine: Clinical tool or research probe? Radiology 170:1–15, 1989.
16. Bradley WG Jr, Tsuruda JS: Perspective: MR sequence parameter optimization: An algorithmic approach. AJR 149:815–823, 1987.
17. Bradley WG: When should GRASS be used? Radiology 169:574–575, 1988.
18. Brant-Zawadzki M, Jeffrey RB Jr, Minagi H, Pitts LH: High resolution CT of thoracolumbar fractures. AJNR 3:69–74, 1982.
19. Brant-Zawadzki M, Norman D (eds): Magnetic Resonance Imaging of the Central Nervous System. New York, Raven Press, 1987.
20. Brodsky AE: Post-laminectomy and post-fusion stenosis of the lumbar spine. Clin Orthop Rel Res 115:130–139, 1976.
21. Brown BM, Schwartz RH, Frank E, Blank NK: Preoperative evaluation of cervical radiculopathy and myelopathy by surface-coil MR imaging. AJR 151:1205–1212, 1988.
22. Bundschuh C, Modic MT, Kearney F, et al: Rheumatoid arthritis of the cervical spine: Surface-coil MR imaging. AJR 151:181–187, 1988.

23. Bundschuh CV, Modic MT, Ross JS, et al: Epidural fibrosis and recurrent disk herniation in the lumbar spine: MR imaging assessment. AJR 150:923–932, 1988.
24. Burton CV, Kirkaldy-Willis WH, Yong-Hing K, Heithoff KB: Causes of failure of surgery on the lumbar spine. Clin Orthop Rel Res 157:191–199, 1981.
25. Bushong SC: Magnetic Resonance Imaging: Physical and Biological Principles. St. Louis, CV Mosby, 1988.
26. Carmody RF, Yang PJ, Seeley GW, et al: Spinal cord compression due to metastatic disease: Diagnosis with MR imaging versus myelography. Radiology 173:225–229, 1989.
27. Carrera GF, Haughton VM, Syvertsen A, Williams AL: Computed tomography of the lumbar facet joints. Radiology 134:145–148, 1980.
28. Chafetz N, Cann CE, Morris JM, et al: Pseudarthrosis following lumbar fusion: Detection by direct coronal CT scanning. Radiology 162:803–805, 1987.
29. Chan F-L, Ho EKW, Chau EMT: Spinal pseudarthrosis complicating ankylosing spondylitis: Comparison of CT and conventional tomography. AJR 150:611–614, 1988.
30. Cohen WA, Maravilla KR, Shuman WP, Dalley RW: Evaluation of metastatic spinal disease with high-field STIR: Comparison of multiple imaging sequences. Radiology 173(P)(suppl):156, 1989.
31. Condon BR, Hadley DM: Quantification of cord deformation and dynamics during flexion and extension of the cervical spine using MR imaging. J Comput Assist Tomogr 12:947–955, 1988.
32. Cooper LS, Chalmers TC, McCally M, et al: The poor quality of early evaluations of magnetic resonance imaging. JAMA 259:3277–3280, 1988.
33. Coventry MB, Ghormley RK, Kernohan JW: The intervertebral disc: Its microscopic anatomy and pathology. Part II. Changes in the intervertebral disc concomitant with age. J Bone Joint Surg 27:233–247, 1945.
34. Daniels DL, Grogan JP, Johansen JG, et al: Cervical radiculopathy: Computed tomography and myelography compared. Radiology 151:109–113, 1984.
35. De La Torre JC: Spinal cord injury. Spine 6:315–335, 1981.
36. Dillin WH, Watkins RG: Cervical myelopathy and cervical radiculopathy. Sem Spine Surg 1:200–208, 1989.
37. Dillon WP, Norman D, Newton TH, et al: Intradural spinal cord lesions: Gadolinium-DTPA-enhanced MR imaging. Radiology 170:229–237, 1989.
38. Dvorak J, Grob D, Baumgartner H, et al: Functional evaluation of the spinal cord by magnetic resonance imaging in patients with rheumatoid arthritis and instability of upper cervical spine. Spine 14:1057–1064, 1989.
39. Edelman RR, Shoukimas GM, Stark DD, et al: High-resolution of surface-coil imaging of lumbar disk disease. AJR 144:1123–1129, 1985.
40. Edelson JG, Nathan H: Nerve root compression in spondylolysis and spondylolisthesis. J Bone Joint Surg 68B:596–599, 1986.
41. Edwards WC, LaRocca H: The developmental segmental sagittal diameter of the cervical spinal canal in patients with cervical spondylosis. Spine 8:20–27, 1983.
42. Emery SE, Pathria MN, Wilber RG, et al: Magnetic resonance imaging of posttraumatic spinal ligament injury. J Spinal Dis 2:229–233, 1989.
43. Enzmann DR, Rubin JB, Wright A: Cervical spine MR imaging: Generating high-signal CSF in sagittal and axial images. Radiology 163:233–238, 1987.
44. Epstein JA, Carras R, Hyman RA, Costa S: Cervical myelopathy caused by developmental stenosis of the spinal canal. J Neurosurg 51:362–367, 1979.
45. Epstein JA, Epstein NE, Marc J, et al: Lumbar intervertebral disk herniation in teenage children: Recognition and management of associated anomalies. Spine 9:427–432, 1984.
46. Erkintalo M, Salminen JJ, Paajanen H, et al: Disk degeneration in 14-year-old children: MR imaging study on low back pain and asymptomatic groups. Radiology 173(P)(suppl):313, 1989.
47. Firooznia H, Benjamin V, Kricheff II, et al: CT of lumbar spine disk herniation: Correlation with surgical findings. AJR 5:91–96, 1984.
48. Forristall RM, Marsh HO, Pay NT: Magnetic resonance imaging and contrast CT of the lumbar spine: Comparison of diagnostic methods and correlation with surgical findings. Spine 13:1049–1054, 1988.
49. Fredericks RK, Elster A, Walker FO: Gadolinium-enhanced MRI: A superior technique for the diagnosis of intraspinal metastases. Neurology 39:734–736, 1989.
50. Fries JW, Abodeely DA, Vijungco JG, et al: Computed tomography of herniated and extruded nucleus pulposus. J Comp Assist Tomogr 6:874–887, 1982.
51. Frocrain L, Duvauferrier R, Husson JL, et al: Recurrent postoperative sciatica: Evaluation with MR imaging and enhanced CT. Radiology 170:531–533, 1989.

52. Frymoyer JW, Newberg A, Pope MH, et al: Spine radiographs in patients with low-back pain. J Bone Joint Surg 66A:1048–1055, 1984.
53. Fujiwara K, Yonenobu K, Ebara S, et al: The prognosis of surgery for cervical compression myelopathy: An analysis of the factors involved. J Bone Joint Surg 71B:393–398, 1989.
54. Fujiwara K, Yonenobu K, Hiroshima K, et al: Morphometry of the cervical spinal cord and its relation to pathology in cases with compression myelopathy. Spine 13:1212–1216, 1988.
55. Gellad FE, Levine AM, Joslyn JN, et al: Pure thoracolumbar facet dislocation: Clinical features and CT appearance. Radiology 161:505–508, 1986.
56. Genant H: Technical considerations. In Newton TH, Potts DG (eds): Computed Tomography of the Spine and Spinal Cord. San Anselmo, CA, Clavadel Press, 1983, pp 1–14.
57. Ghosh P (ed): The Biology of the Intervertebral Disc, Vol I. Boca Raton, FL, CRC Press, 1988.
58. Ghosh P (ed): The Biology of the Intervertebral Disc, Vol II. Boca Raton, FL, CRC Press, 1988.
59. Glenn WV Jr, Rhodes ML, Altschuler EM, et al: Multiplanar display computerized body tomography applications in the lumbar spine. Spine 4:282–294, 1979.
60. Glenn WV Jr, Rothman SLG, Rhodes ML, Kerber CW: An overview of lumbar computed tomography/multiplanar reformations: What are its elements and how do they fit together? In Post MJD (ed): Computed Tomography of the Spine. Baltimore, Williams & Wilkins, 1984, pp 135–154.
61. Goyal RN, Russell NA, Benoit BG, Belanger JMEG: Intraspinal cysts: A classification and literature review. Spine 12:209–213, 1987.
62. Grenier N, Greselle JF, Vital JM, et al: Normal and disrupted lumbar longitudinal ligaments: Correlative MR and anatomic study. Radiology 171:197–205, 1989.
63. Grenier N, Kressel HY, Schiebler ML, Grossman RI: Isthmic spondylolysis of the lumbar spine: MR imaging at 1.5T. Radiology 170:489–493, 1989.
64. Grenier N, Kressel HY, Schiebler ML, et al: Normal and degenerative posterior spinal structures: MR imaging. Radiology 165:517–525, 1987.
65. Grubb SA, Lipscomb HJ, Coonrad RW: Degenerative adult onset scoliosis. Spine 13:241–245, 1988.
66. Gunzburg R, Sandhu A, Fraser RD: The value of computerized tomography in determining lumbar facet joint orientation. J Spinal Dis 2:170–175, 1989.
67. Hansen ST, Taylow TK, Honet JC, Lewis FR: Fracture-dislocations of the ankylosed thoracic spine in rheumatoid spondylitis: Ankylosing spondylitis, Marie-Strumpell disease. J Trauma 7:827–837, 1967.
68. Hashimoto T, Kaneda K, Abumi K: Relationship between traumatic spinal canal stenosis and neurologic deficits in thoracolumbar burst fractures. Spine 13:1268–1272, 1988.
69. Hasso AN, McKinney JM, Killeen J, et al: Computed tomography of children and adolescents with suspected spinal stenosis. J Comput Assist Tomogr 11:609–611, 1987.
70. Hasue M, Kikuchi S, Sakuyama Y, Ito T: Anatomic study of the interrelation between lumbosacral nerve roots and their surrounding tissues. Spine 8:50–57, 1983.
71. Haughton VM, Eldevik OP, Magnaes B, Amundsen P: A prospective comparison of computed tomography and myelography in the diagnosis of herniated lumbar disks. Radiology 142:103–110, 1982.
72. Hedberg MC, Drayer BP, Flom RA, et al: Gradient echo (GRASS) MR imaging in cervical radiculopathy. AJR 150:683–689, 1988.
73. Heiken JP, Glazer HS, Lee JKT, et al: Manual of Clinical Magnetic Resonance Imaging. New York, Raven Press, 1986.
74. Heindel W, Friedmann G, Bunke J, et al: Artifacts in MR imaging after surgical intervention. J Comput Assist Tomogr 10:596–599, 1986.
75. Heithoff KB: Magnetic resonance imaging of the lumbar spine. In Kirkaldy-Willis (ed): Managing Low Back Pain. New York, Churchill Livingstone, 1988, pp 183–208.
76. Herman GT: Three-dimensional imaging on a CT or MR scanner. J Comput Assist Tomogr 12:450–458, 1988.
77. Hickey DS, Aspden RM, Hukins DWL, et al: Analysis of magnetic resonance images from normal and degenerate lumbar intervertebral discs. Spine 11:702–708, 1986.
78. Hochhauser L, Kieffer SA, Cacayorin ED, et al: Recurrent postdiskectomy low back pain: MR-surgical correlation. AJR 151:755–760, 1988.
79. Holt S, Yates PO: Cervical spondylosis and nerve root lesions: Incidence at routine necropsy. J Bone Joint Surg 48B:407–423, 1966.
80. Hueftle MG, Modic MT, Ross JS, et al: Lumbar spine: Postoperative MR imaging with gadolinium-DTPA. Radiology 167:817–824, 1988.

81. Hurme M, Alaranta H: Factors predicting the result of surgery for lumbar intervertebral disc herniation. Spine 12:933–938, 1987.
82. Jaffray D, O'Brien JP: Isolated intervertebral disc resorption: A source of mechanical and inflammatory back pain? Spine 11:397–401, 1986.
83. Johnsson K-E, Willner S, Johnsson K: Postoperative instability after decompression for lumbar spinal stenosis. Spine 11:107–110, 1986.
84. Kambin P, Nixon JE, Chait A, Schaffer JL: Annular protrusion: Pathophysiology and roentgenographic appearance. Spine 13:671–675, 1988.
85. Kawaida H, Sakou T, Morizono Y, Yoshikuni N: Magnetic resonance imaging of upper cervical disorders in rheumatoid arthritis. Spine 14:1144–1148, 1989.
86. Kénési C, Lesur E: Orientation of the articular processes at L4, L5, and S1: Possible role in pathology of the intervertebral disc. Anat Clin 7:43–47, 1985.
87. Kirkaldy-Willis WH: The pathology and pathogenesis of low back pain. In Kirkaldy-Willis WH (ed): Managing Low Back Pain. New York, Churchill Livingstone, 1988, pp 49–75.
88. Kneeland JB, Hyde JS: High-resolution MR imaging with local coils. Radiology 171:1–7, 1989.
89. Kobori M, Takahashi H, Mikawa Y: Atlanto-axial dislocation in Down's syndrome: Report of two cases requiring surgical correction. Spine 11:195–200, 1986.
90. Kortelainen P, Puranen J, Koivisto E, Lahde S: Symptoms and signs of sciatica and their relation to the locaization of the lumbar disc herniation. Spine 10:88–92, 1985.
91. Krol G, Sze G, Malkin M, Walker R: MR of cranial and spinal meningeal carcinomatosis: Comparison with CT and myelography. AJR 151:583–588, 1988.
92. Kulkarni MV, McArdle CB, Kopanicky D, et al: Acute spinal cord injury: MR imaging at 1.5T. Radiology 164:837–843, 1987.
93. Lancourt JE, Glenn WV Jr, Wiltse LL: Multiplanar computerized tomography in the normal spine and in the diagnosis of spinal stenosis: A gross anatomic-computerized tomographic correlation. Spine 4:379–390, 1979.
94. Lauterbur PC: Image formation by induced local interactions: Examples employing nuclear magnetic resonance. Nature 242:190–191, 1973.
95. Lee BCP, Zimmerman RD, Manning JJ, Deck MDF: MR imaging of syringomyelia and hydromyelia. AJR 144:1149–1156, 1985.
96. Lee CK: Lumbar spinal instability (olisthesis) after extensive posterior spinal decompression. Spine 8:429–433, 1983.
97. Lee CK: Accelerated degeneration of the segment adjacent to a lumbar fusion. Spine 13:375–377, 1988.
98. Levitan LH, Wiens CW: Chronic lumbar extradural hematoma: CT findings. Radiology 148:707–708, 1983.
99. Lipson SJ, Muir H: Proteoglycans in experimental intervertebral disc degeneration. Spine 6:194–210, 1981.
100. MacNab I: Spondylolisthesis with an intact neural arch, the so-called pseudo-spondylolistheses. J Bone Joint Surg 32B:325–333, 1950.
101. MacNab I: Cervical spondylosis. Clin Orthop Rel Res 109:69–77, 1975.
102. Maiman DJ, Daniels D, Larson SJ: Magnetic resonance imaging in the diagnosis of lower thoracic disc herniation. J Spinal Disorders 1:134–138, 1988.
103. Maravilla KR, Hartling RP: Imaging decisions in degenerative spinal disease: A practical approach. MRI Decisions 2:2–13, 1988.
104. Maravilla KR, Weinreb JC, Suss R, Nunnally RL: Magnetic resonance demonstration of multiple sclerosis plaques in the cervical cord. AJR 144:381–385, 1985.
105. Mark AS, Atlas SW: MRI of the cervical spine and cord. MRI Decisions May/June:23–32, 1988.
106. Masaryk TJ, Ross JS, Modic MT, et al: High-resolution MR imaging of sequestered lumbar intervertebral disks. AJR 150:1155–1162, 1988.
107. McAfee PC, Ullrich CG, Yuan HA, et al: Computed tomography in degenerative spinal stenosis. Clin Orthop Rel Res 161:221–234, 1981.
108. McAfee PC, Yuan HA, Fredrickson BE, Lubicky JP: The value of computed tomography in thoracolumbar fractures: An analysis of one hundred consecutive cases and a new classification. J Bone Joint Surg 65A:461–473, 1983.
109. Miller JAA, Schmatz C, Schultz AB: Lumbar disc degeneration: Correlation with age, sex, and spine level in 600 autopsy specimens. Spine 13:173–178, 1988.
110. Mink JH: Imaging evaluation of the candidate for percutaneous lumbar discectomy. Clin Orthop Rel Res 238:83–103, 1989.

111. Mirvis SE, Geisler FH, Jelinek JJ, et al: Acute cervical spine trauma: Evaluation with 1.5-T MR imaging. Radiology 166:807–816, 1988.
112. Miyasaka K, Isu T, Iwasaki Y, et al: High resolution computed tomography in the diagnosis of cervical disc disease. Neuroradiology 24:253–257, 1983.
113. Modic MT, Feiglin DH, Piraino DW, et al: Vertebral osteomyelitis: Assessment using MR. Radiology 157:157–166, 1985.
114. Modic MT, Masaryk T, Boumphrey F, et al: Lumbar herniated disk disease and canal stenosis: Prospective evaluation by surface coil MR, CT and myelography. AJR 147:757–765, 1986.
115. Modic MT, Masaryk TJ, Mulopulos GP, et al: Cervical radiculopathy: Prospective evaluation with surface coil MR imaging, CT with metrizamide, and metrizamide myelography. Radiology 161:753–759, 1986.
116. Modic MT, Masaryk TJ, Ross JS: Magnetic Resonance Imaging of the Spine. Chicago, Year Book, 1989.
117. Modic MT, Masaryk TJ, Ross JS, Carter JR: Imaging of degenerative disk disease. Radiology 168:177–186, 1988.
118. Modic MT, Masaryk TJ, Ross JS, et al: Cervical radiculopathy: Value of oblique MR imaging. Radiology 163:227–231, 1987.
119. Modic MT, Ross JS, Masaryk TJ: Imaging of degenerative disease of the cervical spine. Clin Orthop Rel Res 239:109–120, 1989.
120. Modic MT, Steinberg PM, Ross JS, et al: Degenerative disk disease: Assessment of changes in vertebral body marrow with MR imaging. Radiology 166:193–199, 1988.
121. Mooney V, Robertson J: The facet syndrome. Clin Orthop Rel Res 115:149–156, 1976.
122. Nesbit GM, Miller GM, Baker HL Jr, et al: Spinal cord sarcoidosis: A new finding at MR imaging with gadolinium-DTPA enhancement. Radiology 173:839–843, 1989.
123. Norman D, Mills CM, Brant-Zawadzki M, et al: Magnetic resonance imaging of the spinal cord and canal: Potentials and limitations. AJR 141:1147–1152, 1983.
124. O'Callaghan JP, Ullrich CG, Yuan HA, Kieffer SA: CT of facet distraction in flexion injuries of the thoracolumbar spine: The "naked" facet. AJNR 1:97–102, 1980.
125. Paajanen H, Erkintalo M, Kuusela T, et al: Magnetic resonance study of disc degeneration in young low-back pain patients. Spine 14:982–985, 1989.
126. Patronas NJ, Jafar J, Brown F: Pseudomeningoceles diagnosed by metrizamide myelography and computerized tomography. Surg Neurol 16:188–191, 1981.
127. Pavlicek W, Geisinger M, Castle L, et al: The effects of nuclear magnetic resonance on patients with cardiac pacemakers. Radiology 147:149–153, 1983.
128. Pech P, Haughton VM: Lumbar intervertebral disk: Correlative MR and anatomic study. Radiology 156:699–701, 1985.
129. Peck WW: Current status of MRI of the cervical spine. Appl Radiol January:17–30, 1989.
130. Peyster RG, Teplick JG, Haskin M: Computed tomography of lumbosacral conjoined nerve root anomalies: Potential cause of false-positive reading for herniated nucleus-pulposus. Spine 10:331–337, 1985.
131. Porter RW, Hibbert C, Evans C: The natural history of root entrapment syndrome. Spine 9:418–421, 1984.
132. Post MJD, Quencer RM, Montalvo BM, et al: Spinal infection: Evaluation with MR imaging and intraoperative US. Radiology 169:765–771, 1988.
133. Powell MC, Szypryt P, Wilson M, Symonds EM: Prevalence of lumbar disc degeneration observed by magnetic resonance in symptomless women. Lancet ii:1366–1367, 1986.
134. Quencer RM, Sheldon JJ, Post MJD, et al: MRI of the chronically injured cervical spinal cord. AJR 147:125–132, 1986.
135. Raghavan N, Barkovich AJ, Edwards M, Norman D: MR imaging in the tethered spinal cord syndrome. AJR 152:843–852, 1989.
136. Ramsey RG, Zacharias CE: MR imaging of the spine after radiation therapy: Easily recognizable effects. AJR 144:1131–1135, 1985.
137. Rauschning W: Normal and pathologic anatomy of the lumbar root canals. Spine 12:1008–1019, 1987.
138. Reicher MA, Lufkin RB, Smith S, et al: Multiple-angle, variable-interval, nonorthogonal MRI. AJR 147:363–366, 1986.
139. Roberson GH, Llewellyn HJ, Taveras JM: The narrow lumbar spinal canal syndrome. Radiology 107:89–97, 1973.
140. Rosen BR, Fleming DM, Kushner DC, et al: Hematologic bone marrow disorders: Quantitative chemical shift MR imaging. Radiology 169:799–804, 1988.

141. Ross JS, Masaryk TJ, Delamater R, et al: MR imaging of lumbar arachnoiditis. AJR 149:1025–1032, 1987.
142. Ross JS, Masaryk TJ, Modic MT, et al: Lumbar spine: Postoperative assessment with surface-coil MR imaging. Radiology 164:851–860, 1987.
143. Ross JS, Modic MT, Masaryk JJ: Tears of the anulus fibrosus: Assessment with Gd-DTPA-enhanced MR imaging. AJR 154:159–162, 1990.
144. Ross JS, Perez-Reyes N, Masaryk TJ, et al: Thoracic disk herniation: MR imaging. Radiology 165:511–515, 1987.
145. Rothman SLG, Glenn WV Jr: CT multiplanar reconstruction in 253 cases of lumbar spondylolysis. AJNR 5:81–90, 1984.
146. Rothman SLG, Glenn WV Jr: CT evaluation of interbody fusion. Clin Orthop Rel Res 193:47–56, 1985.
147. Rothman SLG, Glenn WV Jr, Kerber CW: Postoperative fractures of lumbar articular facets: Occult cause of radiculopathy. AJR 145:779–784, 1985.
148. Rusinek H, Mourino MR, Firooznia H, et al: Volumetric rendering of MR images. Radiology 171:269–272, 1989.
149. Sato K, Wakamatsu E, Yoshizumi A, et al: The configuration of the laminas and facet joints in degenerative spondylolisthesis: A clinicoradiologic study. Spine 14:1265–1271, 1989.
150. Schaefer DM, Flanders A, Northrup BE, et al: Magnetic resonance imaging of acute cervical spine trauma: Correlation with severity of neurologic injury. Spine 14:1090–1095, 1989.
151. Schnebel B, Kingston S, Watkins R, Dillin W: Comparison of MRI to contrast CT in the diagnosis of spinal stenosis. Spine 14:332–337, 1989.
152. Schneck CD: The anatomy of lumbar spondylosis. Clin Orthop Rel Res 193:20–37, 1985.
153. Sebag GH, Moore SG: Gradient-echo imaging of bone marrow in the appendicular skeleton. Radiology 173(P)(suppl):141, 1989.
154. Shellock FG: MR imgaing of metallic implants and materials: A compilation of the literature. AJR 151:811–814, 1988.
155. Sherry CS, Harms SE, McCroskey WK: Spinal MR imaging: Multiplanar representation from a single high resolution 3D acquisition. J Comput Assist Tomogr 11:859–862, 1987.
156. Simon JH, Szumowski J: Chemical shift imaging with paramagnetic contrast material enhancement for improved lesion depiction. Radiology 171:539–543, 1989.
157. Smith AS, Weinstein MA, Mizushima A, et al: MR imaging characteristics of tuberculous spondylitis vs vertebral osteomyelitis. AJR 153:399–405, 1989.
158. Smith SR, Williams CE, Davies JM, Edwards RHT: Bone marrow disorders: Characterization with quantitative MR imaging. Radiology 172:805–810, 1989.
159. Stanley JH, Schabel SI, Frey GD, Hungerford GD: Quantitative analysis of the cervical spinal canal by computed tomography. Neuroradiology 28:139–143, 1986.
160. Sugimura K, Yamasaki K, Kitagaki H, et al: Bone marrow diseases of the spine: Differentiation with T1 and T2 relaxation times in MR imaging. Radiology 165:541–544, 1987.
161. Sze G, Bravo S, Krol G: Spinal lesions: Quantitative and qualitative temporal evolution of gadopentetate dimeglumine enhancement in MR imaging. Radiology 170:849–856, 1989.
162. Sze G, Krol G, Zimmerman RD, Deck MDF: Intramedullary disease of the spine: Diagnosis using gadolinium-DTPA-enhanced MR imaging. AJR 151:1193–1204, 1988.
163. Sze G, Krol G, Zimmerman RD, Deck MDF: Malignant extradural spinal tumors: MR imaging with gadolinium-DTPA. Radiology 167:217–223, 1988.
164. Szypryt EP, Twining P, Mulholland RC, Worthington BS: The prevalence of disc degeneration associated with neural arch defects of the lumbar spine assessed by magnetic resonance imaging. Spine 14:977–981, 1989.
165. Takahashi M, Yamashita Y, Sakamoto Y, Kojima R: Chronic cervical cord compression: Clinical significance of increased signal intensity on MR images. Radiology 173:219–224, 1989.
166. Teitelbaum GP, Bradley WG Jr, Klein BD: MR imaging artifacts, ferromagnetism, and magnetic torque of intravascular filters, stents, and coils. Radiology 166:657–664, 1988.
167. Teresi LM, Lufkin RB, Reicher MA, et al: Asymptomatic degenerative disk disease and spondylosis of the cervical spine: MR imaging. Radiology 164:83–88, 1987.
168. Teresi LM, Lufkin RL, Hanafee WN: MRI of the cervical spine. Appl Radiol August:31–44, 1988.
169. Tracy PT, Wright RM, Hanigan WC: Magnetic resonance imaging of spinal injury. Spine 14:292–301, 1989.
170. Van Lom KJ, Kellerhouse LE, Pathria MN, et al: Infection versus tumor in the spine: Criteria for distinction with CT. Radiology 166:851–855, 1988.
171. Van Schaik JPJ, Verbiest H, Van Schaik FDJ: The orientation of laminae and facet joints in the lower lumbar spine. Spine 10:59–63, 1985.

172. VanDyke C, Ross JS, Tkach J, et al: Gradient-echo MR imaging of the cervical spine: Evaluation of extradural disease. AJR 153:393–398, 1989.
173. Verbiest H: Fallacies of the present definition, nomenclature, and classification of the stenosis of the lumbar vertebral canal. Spine 1:217–225, 1976.
174. Verbiest H: Words, images, knowledge, and reality: Some reflections from the neurosurgical perspective. Acta Neurochirugica 69:163–193, 1983.
175. Vogler JB III, Murphy WA: Bone marrow imaging. Radiology 168:679–693, 1988.
176. Weinreb JC, Wolbarsht LB, Cohen JM, et al: Prevalence of lumbosacral intervertebral disk abnormalities on MR images in pregnant and asymptomatic nonpregnant women. Radiology 170:125–128, 1989.
177. Wiesel SW, Tsourmas N, Feffer HL, et al: A study of computer-assisted tomography. I. The incidence of positive CAT scans in an asymptomatic group of patients. Spine 9:549–556, 1984.
178. Williams AL, Haughton VM, Meyer GA, Ho KC: Computed tomographic appearance of the bulging annulus. Radiology 142:403–408, 1982.
179. Williams AL, Haughton VM, Pojunas KW, et al: Differentiation of intramedullary neoplasms and cysts by MR. AJR 149:159–164, 1987.
180. Williams MP, Cherryman GR, Husband JE: Significance of thoracic disc herniation demonstrated by MR imaging. J Comput Assist Tomogr 13:211–214, 1989.
181. Wiltse L: Far-out syndrome. In Rothman SLG, Glenn WV Jr (eds): Multiplanar CT of the Spine. Baltimore, University Park Press, 1985.
182. Wiltse LL, Widell EH Jr, Jackson DW: Fatigue fracture: The basic lesion in isthmic spondylolisthesis. J Bone Joint Surg 57A:17, 1975.
183. Wozney P, Jacobson MS, Zimmermann RT: A systems approach to computed tomographic image quality. In Post MJD (ed): Computed Tomography of the Spine. Baltimore, Williams & Wilkins, 1984, pp 119–134.
184. Yu S, Haughton VM, Ho PSP, et al: Progressive and regressive changes in the nucleus pulposus: Part II. The adult. Radiology 169:93–97, 1988.
185. Yu S, Haughton VM, Sether LA, et al: Criteria for classifying normal and degenerated lumbar intervertebral disks. Radiology 170:523–526, 1989.
186. Yu S, Sether LA, Ho PSP, et al: Tears of the anulus fibrosus: Correlation between MR and pathologic findings in cadavers. AJNR 9:367–370, 1988.
187. Zucherman J, Derby R, Hsu K, et al: Normal magnetic resonance imaging with abnormal discography. Spine 13:1355–1359, 1988.

MARK J. SONTAG, MD

FUNCTIONAL ASSESSMENT OF THE SPINAL PAIN PATIENT

From the San Francisco Spine
  Institute
Daly City, California

Reprint requests to:
Mark J. Sontag, MD
San Francisco Spine Institute
1850 Sullivan Avenue, #140
Daly City, CA 94015

Historically, diagnosing and treating patients have been the cornerstones of medicine. Currently, the quality of a patient's life and the functional outcome of treatment are also thought to be of paramount importance. In the diagnosis and treatment of musculoskeletal injuries, the functional assessment of peripheral joints is an accepted practice. Recently, approaches and evaluating tools used in the diagnosis and treatment of musculoskeletal injuries have been applied to the spine patient. This chapter discusses the importance and current status of the functional assessment of the patient with spinal pain.

THE NECESSITY OF FUNCTIONAL ASSESSMENT OF THE SPINE PATIENT

Low back pain alone affects approximately 85% of all persons in the Western world at some point during their lives.[9] Low back pain is second only to upper respiratory infections as the most frequent reason why individuals seek medical attention. It is the most frequent cause of activity limitation and disability in persons under age 45 years and the third most frequent cause in the 45 to 64 year old age group.[5]

Approximately 2% of all workers injure their backs annually.[17] Although the majority of low back pain sufferers improve within 3 months, the costs still exceed 16 billion dollars each year.[80] Incredibly, 10% of the injuries represent 80% of the total costs.[82] It is estimated that 50% of individuals disabled due to low back pain have absolutely no objective findings.[63,85]

Exorbitant amounts of money are spent for a small percentage of low back sufferers who have very few objective abnormalities. The economic magnitude of this problem has prompted investigators to try to objectify spinal function and dysfunction in an attempt to quantitate true abnormalities. Due to the complexity of the spine and large discrepancies among spinal diagnoses, practicing clinicians have often relied completely on a patient's subjective complaints. Recently, an attempt has been made to evaluate low back pain patients functionally rather than subjectively. Cerebrovascular scales, for instance, concentrate on an individual's function and not on subjective complaints of pain. Evans and Kagan[31] have developed a functional rating scale for chronic low back patients that quantifies the patient's level of activity and relative personal independence. Deyo recently reviewed current techniques that measure functional status, and their usefulness.[29]

THE POTENTIAL BENEFITS OF FUNCTIONAL ASSESSMENT

Currently an inordinate amount of importance is placed on subjective complaints and not enough attention is given to objective findings or functional parameters. Functional assessment of spine patients includes an objective analysis of their condition and of their subsequent recovery. Objective analysis of the spine allows one to determine deficits and conceivably correct them more rapidly. In addition, assessments of multiple aspects of spinal function will increase biomechanical understanding of the spine and psychological information about the patient with spinal disorders. Functional assessment of the spine might validate the qualified injured worker and identify the malingerer or individual whose complaints are influenced by issues of secondary gain. Functional testing should reassure workers that they are indeed able and capable of performing the tasks required by their jobs prior to returning to the actual job site. Once normative data have been obtained and the predictiveness of the testing has been established, then preplacement screening might be instituted as a means of actually preventing injuries.

SPINE PAIN PREVENTION AND SCREENING

Future benefits of standardized functional assessment of the spine include earlier return to work and reduced disability costs following an injury. These economic results would directly benefit patients, employers, insurance companies, and the consumer.

Historically, preemployment histories and physical examinations have been used to screen potential employees.[6] Although it has been established that a previous history of low back pain predisposes an individual to additional low back pain,[24] prospective employees have been known to distort their own histories to facilitate employment. Rowe estimates that only 7 to 8% of individuals prone to developing low back pain can be screened via the preemployment history and physical examination.[75] However, Chaffin et al.[24] and Snook et al.[79] were unable to identify susceptible workers using preplacement examinations.

In the 1950s and 1960s, preplacement radiographs of the lumbar spine gained acceptance.[16,37,60] However, other studies have concluded that preemployment radiographs alone are not predictive of future low back injury.[51,62,70,72] Recently, Frymoyer et al. have demonstrated an association between low back pain and radiographic L4–5 disc space narrowing and spurs.[33] Current research is investigating the relationship between lumbar spinal canal diameter and the likelihood of low back pain.[69] Saal and Saal[75] have demonstrated that those individuals with herniated nucleus pulposus that do not respond to nonoperative treatment are likely to have concomitant spinal stenosis. Thus, although plain radiographs are not predictive of low back injury, it is possible that spinal canal diameter might be a predictive factor.

Anthropometric measurements (e.g., height, weight, and body frame) have not been predictive of subsequent low back injury.[25,36,72] Psychological factors certainly play a role in recovery from low back injury; however, they are not good predictors of the development of low back pain.

The three current approaches to risk management of spinal injuries in the work place include (1) ergonomic changes, (2) preplacement or preselection screening, and (3) education and training for employees. Snook defined ergonomics as "designing the job to fit the capabilities and limitations of the worker."[81] Analyzing the three approaches mentioned above, Snook et al.[79] found that only ergonomic changes in the work place were actually successful in reducing injuries. They found that preplacement screening and education were not successful. Ergonomic changes are certainly successful in reducing low back injuries, yet they are often cumbersome and expensive to incorporate into our current work place.

Preplacement screening is currently very appealing to employers. Rather than designing the work site for the worker, employers attempt to select workers who can be productive at a given work site. The preselection process is often based on strength determinations. The various techniques for evaluating strength will be discussed later in this chapter. The most common approach used in an attempt to reduce injuries in the work place is education and training. The education often consists of in-house instruction in proper lifting and bending techniques. The success of these in-house programs has not be scientifically established.[27,79]

Biomechanical studies have offered great insight into the stresses and torque placed on the lumbar spine in individuals involved in manual material handling.[23] Andersson has demonstrated that the distance an object is from the body influences the stress upon the spine more than the actual lifting method.[4] There remains significant controversy in the scientific literature about the proper way to actually lift. Physiologic studies have suggested a relationship between low back injury and muscular fatigue.[23] Additional prospective studies are needed to evaluate the efficacy of biomechanical and physiologic methodologies.

SPINE PAIN IN INDUSTRY

To successfully analyze and objectively measure spinal function, one must understand the multifactorial nature of spine injury. Spine injury should be analyzed on the basis of physical factors as well as psychosocial factors. Neither group of factors solely addresses the complexity of spinal disability, and therefore both must be considered in unison. In an attempt to quantify spinal function, one must also incorporate the patient's personal perception of his or her physical abilities. Often there is a wide dichotomy between what an individual can actually perform and the perception of such.

Epidemiological data point to lifting as one physical factor that correlates with over 33% of low back injuries.[42] Lifting places a compressive load on the intervertebral disc. White et al. reported that workers' spines that are exposed to compression greater than 6000 newtons have an eight-times higher incidence of low back injuries than those individuals who are exposed to a compression of 3500 newtons.[88] The frequency of lifting is also related to low back injury. Workers who lift most frequently are more likely to be injured.[86] The amount of weight lifted also appears to correlate with the development of low back pain.[36,73,89] Jobs that require lifting greater than 25 pounds are associated with an increased risk of low back injury.[1,2] There appears to be a definite relationship between the development of low back pain and the amount of lifting required in a specific occupation. Workers in heavy industry, nurses, and truck drivers must all lift frequently. Therefore, it is not surprising that these are the professions with the highest prevalence of low back disability.[38]

Magora correlated sudden maximum physical efforts characterized by their unexpectedness to the development of low back pain.[53] He hypothesized that an unexpected sudden maximum motion is more likely to injure the spine than a controlled rehearsed motion.

Improper lifting is the most frequent cause of low back injury.[14] Vibrational exposure and static work postures have also been correlated with the development of low back pain.[33]

The determinants of lifting technique are multifactorial. Manual material handling requires coordination, proprioception, training, experience, intelligence, flexibility of the extremities and spine, strength of the extremities and trunk, and finally endurance.

Psychosocial factors play a tremendous role in spine disability and recovery. The retrospective Boeing Aircraft Employee Study found a correlation between the reports of back injury and poor employee appraisal ratings performed by the employees' supervisors 6 months prior to injury.[15] Magora demonstrated that employees not satisfied with their occupation, place of employment, or social status had a higher incidence of low back pain than control subjects. He also demonstrated that individuals that perceive a high degree of responsibility and mental concentration at work, resulting in a feeling of tenseness and fatigue, were also more likely to develop low back pain.[53] Deyo and Diehl report that psychosocial and demographic features such as education, number of prior episodes of back pain, and whether or not a patient "always feels sick" correlated with low back pain outcome better than physical parameters such as presenting physical examination or the type of physical therapy the patients underwent.[28]

Programs directed at altering management's perspective of the injured worker have been successful in reducing low back injury costs. The Chelsea Back Program consisted of structural, technological, and attitudinal changes of management and resulted in a 75% reduction in the total cost per back injury claim.[32] Wood compared a management attitudinal program with a back school program in back injury prevention. Interestingly, the management attitudinal program was successful in reducing injuries, whereas the back school program had no effect.[88]

The functional task of lifting consists of multiple components, one of which includes strength.[40] Increased abdominal and trunk strength have been correlated with improved outcome following low back injury.[43,47,52] In the next section of this chapter the techniques of quantifying lumbar trunk strength and their relationship to the prediction of future low back pain are evaluated. Table 1 summarizes the multiple factors affecting the manual material handling activities.

TABLE 1. Factors Affecting Manual Materials Handling Activities*

Work Variables	Task Variables	Environmental Variables
Physical factors: Age, sex, anthrometry strength, etc.	The load: Mass, size, shape stability, coupling, etc.	Heat load Noise
Physiological factors: Aerobic power, anaerobic power, endurance, etc.	The workplace: Space, obstacles, etc. Temporal aspects	Vibration Work surface: Geometry, stability, traction, etc.
Training and experience	Complexity	

* From Ayoub MM, et al: Development of strength and capacity norms for manual materials handling activities: The state of the art. Hum Factors 22:271–283, 1980, with permission.

TECHNIQUES OF EVALUATING STRENGTH

There are three common methods of evaluating strength: (1) isometric, (2) isokinetic, and (3) isoinertial (psychophysical). Isometric strength is defined as the static measure of maximum voluntary contraction with the muscle at a fixed length. Isokinetic strength is defined as a dynamic measure with body segments moving at a constant rate of speed. Isoinertial (psychophysical) strength is defined as a dynamic measure of maximum weight moved through a range. The following six criteria can be used to evaluate the above techniques.

1. Test safety
2. Reliability and reproducibility
3. Practicality of test administration
4. Risk factor/predictability
5. Specificity to job requirements
6. Ethically and legally defensible methods.[20]

Isometric Strength Testing

There are currently two basic techniques used in evaluating isometric strength. The first technique can be described as a "low"-technology approach using a simple strain gauge, whereas the "high"-technology approach uses computerized equipment such as Cybex (Lumex Corp., Ronkonkoma, NY), Kin-Com (Chatteck Corp., Chattanooga, TN), Biodex (Biodex, Inc., Shirley, NY) or Lido (Loredan, Inc., Davis, CA) instrumentation. Figure 1 illustrates an isometric strength testing device using a strain gauge. The strain gauge apparatus costs approximately $300, whereas the high-tech computerized equipment is generally more costly.

The reliability and reproducibility of isometric strength testing have been established.[48] One major concern with isometric testing is the safety of the actual procedure. Hansson et al., using biomechanical analysis, have calculated compressive loads on the L3 vertebral body ranging from 5,000 to 11,000 newtons during squat and torso lifting with isometric testing.[34] In vitro, these loads have caused structural failure of the vertebral endplates. Hansson et al. noted, however, that isometric testing of trunk flexors and extensors caused significantly less load on the L3 vertebral body. Zeh et al. analyzed over 1,000 volunteers testing isometric strength.[89] Approximately 5% of the subjects could not continue testing secondary to pain, and 0.5% of the individuals actually developed an injury. Zeh et al.'s recommendation was to reduce the number of

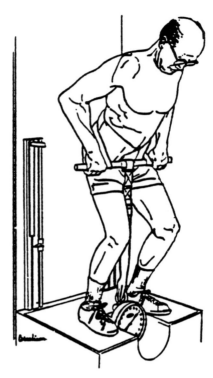

FIGURE 1. An isometric strength measurement. (From Cady LD, et al: Strength and fitness and subsequent back injuries in firefighters. J Occup Med 21:269–272, 1979, with permission.)

exertions, which they found substantially reduced the probability of injury and still provided accurate assessment of an individual's isometric strength. Overall, isometric testing techniques, particularly using the strain gauge devices are quite simple, safe, and practical to administer.

Chaffin and Park first demonstrated that the incidence rate of low back pain is correlated with increased lifting strength requirements.[25] In a subsequent study, Chaffin demonstrated that the incidence of back pain increased when loads exceeded an individual's isometric lifting capability.[21,22,25] On the basis of these data, Chaffin and co-workers demonstrated a reduction in low back injuries by selecting workers on the basis of their isometric strength and placing them in jobs where their strength exceeded their lifting requirements.[44,45] However, Battie et al. have found no correlation between isometric strength and injury, yet they did not match job demands with strength.[8] Considering there is no demonstrated significant difference in static back extensor strength among workers performing a wide variety of physically demanding jobs,[40] isometric strength testing might be a useful tool in preplacing workers.

Isokinetic Strength Testing

There are four commercially available isokinetic testing devices: Cybex provides a sagittal strength device as well as a torsional strength device. Kin-Com markets an attachment to its extremity dynamometer so that it can be used as a back testing device. Biodex systems are similar to the Kin-Com units in that they also provide an attachment to their existing extremity system. Loredan provides a sagittal strength tester similar to the Cybex unit, but allows individuals to sit or stand. Mayer and Gatchel have published excellent review of the above manufacturers' equipment.[55]

The move toward isokinetic trunk muscle testing has arisen from the premise that dynamic testing can more accurately recreate functional lifting than static testing. This premise, however, has not yet been scientifically validated. Also, individuals do not actually lift items isokinetically, but rather isoinertially. Computerized isokinetic technology represents a fixed constrained system that does not represent how an individual actually lifts. However, isokinetic testing has been proved to be safe and the data reproducible and reliable.[26,30,49,50,78,83]

Another popular aspect of isokinetic testing is curve analysis. Hypothetically the curve variability distinguishes submaximal from maximal efforts in isokinetic trunk and lift testing. It is assumed that with accurate and reproducible computerized strength testing, one can distinguish malingering from maximal voluntary effort. Hazard et al. evaluated the variability of isokinetic curves as an indicator of effort.[35] They concluded that clinical observation of the subject using the isokinetic equipment is more accurate than analyzing curve variability. They found it difficult to discriminate between submaximal effort secondary to pain, malingering, or fatigue.

In summary, isokinetic technology is safe and provides repeatable, reproducible data. It is costly technology. Scientific validation has to this date not demonstrated that isokinetic testing is superior to isometric testing procedures. Additionally, it is not job-specific during a rehabilitation program. These factors make it difficult to justify the expense of isokinetic testing versus the lower cost alternative of isometric testing.

Use of isokinetic technologies during a rehabilitation program facilitate recovery from low back injuries,[57] probably due to positive reinforcement. However, the use of isokinetic exercise equipment for rehabilitation purposes is a separate issue and is not covered in this chapter.

Isoinertial Strength Testing

There are two basic approaches to isoinertial strength testing, a low-technology and a high-technology approach. Snook introduced the first strength evaluation using a low-technology isoinertial approach. This involved lifting boxes filled with lead shot or bricks. More recently Mayer et al. have introduced a progressive isoinertial lifting evaluation (Pile).[58,59] In the high-technology arena, the B-100 or B-200 (Isotechnologies, Hillsboro, NC) provides a computerized isoinertial testing device.

The data from the low-tech and high-tech approaches are repeatable and reproducible.[68] The technology is safe to administer and relatively easy to use, particularly the low-technology. The cost for Snook's or Mayer's low technology approaches is low, whereas the cost for the B-100 or B-200 is high. However, isoinertial testing can be job-specific. The multiaxial uncontrolled speed evaluation most closely replicates functional motion of the spine.[67] Unfortunately, the testing data have been demonstrated to be poor predictors of future low back pain.[84]

It has been demonstrated that using high-tech isoinertial testing can reduce low back disability time.[76] It is likely that the reduced disability time associated

TABLE 2.   States of Whole-body Strength Testing*

Criterion	Isometric	Isokinetic	Isoinertial
Repeatable	Excellent	Excellent	Excellent
Safe	Good	Excellent	Excellent
Easy to Use	Excellent	Excellent	Good
Cost	Medium	High	Low
Job-related	Good	?	Good for Lifting
Predictive	Good	?	?

* From Gary Herrin, University of Michigan Center for Ergonomics, Ann Arbor, MI, 1990.

with using both isokinetic and isoinertial high technology is related to the actual objectification of function. By objectifying function, the patient has a direct feedback about his recovery, which most likely serves as a motivator.

Table 2 summarizes the six criteria by which whole-body, strength-testing devices have been judged. It is clear that all of them are relatively safe, easy to use, and provide reproducible data.[10] Only isometric and isoinertial techniques are actually job-related. Most importantly, only isometric strength testing appears to be predictive of future low back injury.

STRENGTH VERSUS ENDURANCE
Do low back pain sufferers sustain their injury due to weak trunk muscles or do they develop muscular weakness after the injury? Many studies have demonstrated that individuals with low back pain have weaker trunk muscles when tested isometrically.[3,41,46,61] Other reports note that low back pain sufferers have weaker trunk muscles when tested dynamically.[56,57,66,77] However, Berkson et al. and Nachemson and Lindh report that there is no difference in isometric abdominal or trunk strength in those individuals with low back pain when compared with age-matched controls.[11,64]

Biering-Sorensen has stated that trunk strength alone is a poor predictor of low back pain.[12,13] However, Biering-Sorensen has demonstrated that isometric back endurance is significant for predicting the first back pain occurrence in men.[13] Nicolaisen and Jorgensen found no difference in abdominal and back strength in back pain patients versus normals.[39,65] However, they did find decreased endurance of the trunk muscles in low back pain sufferers. Reduced endurance in the trunk musculature might force the spine to perform functional activities in an uncoupled, unprotected manner, making injuries more likely.

It is quite obvious that there is extensive controversy about the relationship between trunk strength and low back injury. Based on a critical review of the literature, Chaffin's concept of matching the strength of workers to the strength demands of their jobs based on pure isometric strength testing still carries tremendous merit. Additional investigation in isometric strength versus isometric endurance needs to be explored in light of the data presented in recent studies.

NECK AND UPPER EXTREMITY TESTING DEVICES
There are numerous testing devices that can evaluate various upper extremity parameters in a safe, reliable, reproducible, and practical manner. These devices often recreate functional activities required at the work place or home. In addition to objective performance data, the examiner can observe spinal mechanics and record the consistency of subjective complaints.

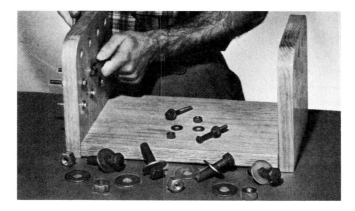

FIGURE 2.   Bennett Hand-tool Dexterity Test. (From 1989 Catalog, The Psychological Corp., Harcourt Brace Jovanovich, Inc., San Diego, CA, 1989, with permission.)

Neck patients often describe subjective difficulty using their hands secondary to neck pain, weakness (radiculopathy), degeneration, or incoordination. Hand dexterity is vital in the majority of work tasks. The following tests all objectify manual speed and dexterity in a safe, reliable, reproducible, and practical manner: Minnesota Rate of Manipulation, O'Connor Tweezer, Bennett Hand-Tool (Fig. 2), Purdue Peg Board, and Jebson Hand-Function. The purchase prices range from $150 to $500. Although these testing devices are job-related, they have not been used to predict injuries.

Work-simulation and work-tolerance tests have been successful in objectifying neck and upper extremity function. The Valpar (Valpar International, Tucson, AZ) testing equipment assesses upper extremity/neck range of motion, eye-hand-foot coordination, form perception, and fatigue. The Work Capacity Evaluation Devices (WEST, Long Beach, CA) functionally determine whole-body range of motion under load lifting and lowering tolerance. The Loredan Upper Cycle Ergonometer (Loredan Biomedical, Davis, CA), measures cardiovascular fitness and endurance while assessing upper extremity strength and range of motion. The Valpar, WEST, and Loredan equipment are all safe, reliable, reproducible, job-related, and practical, yet these devices have not scientifically been demonstrated as predictors of injury.

The BTE Work Simulator (Baltimore Therapeutic Equipment, Hanover, MD) is a versatile device that can simulate numerous work demands at a controlled effort level (cost $25,000). Matheson advocates the use of maximum voluntary effort testing provided by the BTE Work Simulator as a means of identifying the symptom magnifier.[54] He believes that repetitive trials administered maximally over a short period of time will yield consistent results (low coefficient of variation). Inconsistent results (high coefficient of variation) would suggest symptom magnification. The JAMAR Hand Dynamometer (J.A. Preston Corp., Clifton, NJ) is the traditional upper extremity testing device that measures full hand-gripping strength, relying on maximum voluntary effort. The BTE Work Simulator and JAMAR Hand Dynamometer are both safe, reliable, reproducible, job-related, and practical, yet have not scientifically been demonstrated as predictors of injury.

MEDICAL/LEGAL ASPECTS OF EVALUATIONS

In the state of California it is against the law to perform discriminative hiring based on the latent or potential disability. To successfully reject an applicant for a job on the basis of a potential back problem, the following criteria must be fulfilled: (1) inability of the applicant to do the specific job, (2) all or substantially all of the excluded individuals are unable to safely and efficiently perform the job, and (3) there is an identifiable and substantial immediate danger imposing a substantial degree of risk. Chaffin's techniques using isometric strength testing and matching a worker's job to his actual lifting capabilities once the individual is hired are legally defensible.

FUTURE APPLICATION OF FUNCTIONAL ASSESSMENT

Cady's classic description of firefighters demonstrated that the most physically fit individuals had the least number of low back injuries. The prospective measurements included flexibility, isometric lifting strength, bicycle ergometer exercise measurements of 2-minute recovery heart rate, diastolic blood pressure at a heart rate of 60 beats per minute, and watts effort required to sustain heart rate at 160 beats per minute.[19] In a follow-up study, Cady et al. demonstrated that following a 14-year program promoting health and physical fitness, there was a 16% increase in physical work capacity, a slight increase in spinal flexibility, no clear increase in muscle strength, a decrease in smoking, a decrease in disabling injuries, and a 25% decrease in workers' compensation costs.[18] Cady's demonstration of decreased workers' compensation injury and costs using a physical fitness program, Chaffin's demonstration of reduced injuries using isometric testing, and management approaches described previously, all suggest that there are active ways that modern industry can reduce the incidents of spine pain and subsequent compensation. In the future, workers could be better trained and conditioned, and more appropriately matched to their jobs. If the worker is not properly matched to the job, active training or conditioning could be initiated, or an alternative job found.

CONCLUSION

In summary, evaluating spine injury is a complicated problem affected by a myriad of physical, psychosocial, and legal issues. To focus on only one variable, such as strength, results in a gross simplification of this challenging problem. It is quite apparent that industry requires uniformity in testing of the multitude of variables. It also appears that emphasis placed on objective parameters appears to facilitate recovery from a spine injury. Objectification of function is an important goal in rehabilitative medicine. Ergonomic changes, preselection of the worker, and more informed management appear to be the prerequisites for reducing spine pain in the industry. Generalized improved fitness also appears to be very promising. Certainly, additional research and standardization are required in all of these areas.

REFERENCES

1 Adams MA, Hutton WC: The relevance of torsion to the mechanical derangement of the lumbar spine. Spine 6:241–248, 1981.
2. Adams MA, Hutton WC: Prolapsed intervertebral disc: A hyperflexion injury. Spine 7:184–191, 1982.
3. Alston W, et al: A quantitative study of muscle factors in the chronic low back syndrome. J Am Geriatr Soc 14:1041–1047, 1966.

4. Andersson GBJ: Quantitative studies of back loads in lifting. Spine 1:178–185, 1976.
5. Andersson GBJ: Low-back pain in industry. Spine 6:53–56, 1981.
6. Ayoub MA: Control of manual lifting hazards. III. Pre-employment screening. J Occup Med 24:751–761, 1982.
7. Ayoub MM, Mital A, Bakken GM, et al: Development of strength and capacity norms for manual materials handling activities: The state of the art. Hum Factors 22:271–283, 1980.
8. Battie MC, et al: Isometric lifting strength as a predictor of industrial back pain reports. Spine 14:851–856, 1989.
9. Beals RK, Hickman NW: Industrial injuries of the back and extremities. J Bone Joint Surg 54A:1593–1611, 1972.
10. Beimborn D, Morrissey M: A review of the literature related to trunk muscle performance. Spine 13:655–660, 1988.
11. Berkson M, Schultz A, Nachemson A, Andersson G: Voluntary strengths of male adults with acute low back syndrome. Clin Orthop Rel Res 129:84–94, 1977.
12. Biering-Sorensen F: Low back trouble in a general population of 30, 40, 50 and 60-year-old men and women. Dan Med Bull 29:289–299, 1982.
13. Biering-Sorensen F: Physical measurements as risk indicators for low-back trouble over a one-year period. Spine 9:106–119, 1984.
14. Bigos SJ, et al: Back injuries in industry: A retrospective study. II. Injury factors. Spine 11:246–251, 1986.
15. Bigos SJ, et al: Back injuries in industry: A retrospective study. III. Employee-related factors. Spine 11:252–256, 1986.
16. Bond MB: Low-back x-rays. J Occup Med 6:373–380, 1964.
17. Bond MB: Low back injuries in industry. Ind Med Surg 39:28–32, 1970.
18. Cady LD, et al: Program for increasing health and physical fitness of firefighters. J Occup Med 27:110–114, 1985.
19. Cady LD, Bischoff DP, et al: Strength and fitness and subsequent back injuries in firefighters. J Occup Med 21:269–272, 1979.
20. Chaffin DB: Ergonomics guide for the assessment of human static strength. Am Ind Hyg Assoc J 36:505–511, 1975.
21. Chaffin DB: Human strength capability and low-back pain. J Occup Med 16:248–254, 1974.
22. Chaffin DB: Preemployment strength testing: An updated position. J Occup Med 20:403–408, 1978.
23. Chaffin DB: Manual materials handling: The cause of over-exertion injury and illness in industry. J Environ Path Toxicol 2:31–66, 1979.
24. Chaffin DB, Herrin GD, Keyersling WM: Pre-employment strength testing in selecting workers for materials handling jobs. NIOSH CDC 99:62–74, 1976.
25. Chaffin DB, Park KS: A longitudinal study of low-back pain as associated with occupational weight lifting factors. Am Ind Hyg Assoc J 34:513, 1983.
26. Davies GJ: Trunk testing using a prototype Cybex II isokinetic dynamometer stabilization system. JOSPT 3:164–170, 1982.
27. Dedobbeleer N, German P: Safety practices in construction industry. J Occup Med 29:863–868, 1987.
28. Deyo RA, Diehl AK: Predicting disability in patients with low back pain (abstract). Clin Res 34:814A, 1986.
29. Deyo RA: Measuring the functional status of patients with low back pain. Arch Phys Med Rehabil 69:1044–1053, 1988.
30. Elliott J: Assessing muscle strength isokinetically. JAMA 240:2408–2409, 1978.
31. Evans JH: The development of a functional rating scale to measure the treatment outcome of chronic spinal patients. Spine 11:277–281, 1986.
32. Fitzler SL: Attitudinal change: The Chelsea Back Program. Occup Health Saf 51:24–26, 1982.
33. Frymoyer JW, et al: Risk factors in low-back pain. J Bone Joint Surg 65A:213–217, 1983.
34. Hansson TH, et al: The load on the lumbar spine during isometric strength testing. Spine 9:720–724, 1984.
35. Hazard R, Reid S, et al: Isokinetic trunk and lifting strength measurements: Variability as an indicator of effort. Spine 13:54–57, 1988.
36. Hult L: Cervical, dorsal, and lumbar spinal syndromes. Acta Orthop Scand 17:1–102, 1954.
37. Hurley WJ: Lost time back injuries: Their relationship to heavy work and preplacement back x-rays. J Occup Med 14:611–614, 1972.
38. Jensen RC: Epidemiology of work-related back pain. Topics in Acute Care and Trauma Rehabilitation for Industrial Back Injuries, Part I. 2(3):1–17, 1988.

39. Jorgensen K, Nicolaisen T: Trunk extensor endurance: Determination and relation to low-back trouble. Ergonomics 30:259–267, 1987.
40. Kamon E, Goldfuss AJ: In-plant evaluation of the muscle strength of workers. Am Ind Hyg Assoc J 39:801–807, 1978.
41. Karvonen MJ, et al: Back and leg complaints in relation to muscle strength in young men. Scand J Rehabil Med 12:53–59, 1980.
42. Kelsey J, et al: An epidemiologic study of lifting and twisting on the job and risk for acute prolapsed lumbar intervertebral disc. J Orthop Res 2:61–66, 1984.
43. Kendall HP, Jenkins JM: Exercises for backache: A double-blind controlled study. Physiotherapy 53:154–159, 1968.
44. Keyserling WM: Establishing an industrial strength testing program. Am Ind Hyg Assoc J 41:730–736, 1980.
45. Keyserling WM: Isometric strength testing as a means of controlling medical incidents on strenuous jobs. J Occup Med 22:332–336, 1980.
46. Kishino ND, et al: Quantification of lumbar function. Part 4: Isometric and isokinetic lifting simulation in normal subjects and low-back dysfunction patients. Spine 10:921–927, 1985.
47. Kraus H, Nagler W: Evaluation of an exercise program for back pain. AFP 28(3):153–158, 1983.
48. Kroemer KHE: Testing individual capability to lift material: Repeatability of a dynamic test compared with static testing. J Saf Res 16:1–7, 1985.
49. Langrana NA, Lee CK: Isokinetic evaluation of trunk muscles. Spine 9:171–175, 1984.
50. Langranada NA, et al: Quantitative assessment of back strength using isokinetic testing. Spine 9:287–290, 1984.
51. LaRocca H, MacNab I: Value of pre-employment radiographic assessment of the lumbar spine. Can Med Assoc J 101:49–54, 1969.
52. Lidstrom A, Zachrisson M: Physical therapy on low back pain and sciatica. Scand J Rehabil Med 2:37–42, 1970.
53. Magora A: Investigation of the relation between low back pain and occupation. Scand J Rehabil Med 5:186–190, 1973.
54. Matheson LN: Use of the BTE Work Simulator to screen for symptom magnification syndrome. Ind Rehab 2(2): 1989.
55. Mayer T, Gatchel R: Functional Restoration for Spinal Disorders: The Sports Medicine Approach. Philadelphia, Lea & Febiger, 1988, pp 139–161.
56. Mayer TG: Quantification of lumbar function. Part 2. Sagittal plane trunk strength in chronic low-back pain patients. Spine 10:765–772, 1985.
57. Mayer TG, et al: Objective assessment of spine function following industrial injury: A prospective study with comparison group and one-year follow-up. Spine 10:482–493, 1985.
58. Mayer TG, Barnes D, et al: Progressive isoinertial lifting evaluation. II. A comparison with isokinetic lifting in a disabled chronic low-back pain industrial population. Spine 13:998–1002, 1988.
59. Mayer TG, Barnes D, et al: Progressive isoinertial lifting evaluation. I. A standardized protocol and normative database. Spine 13:993–997, 1988.
60. McGill CM: Industrial back problems: A control program. J Occup Med 10:174–178, 1968.
61. McNeil T, et al: Trunk strength in attempted flexion, extension, and lateral bending in healthy subjects and patients with low-back disorders. Spine 5:529–538, 1980.
62. Montgomery CH: Preemployment back x-rays. J Occup Med 18:495–498, 1976.
63. Nachemson A: Work for all. Clin Orthop Rel Res 179:77–82, 1983.
64. Nachemson A, Lindh M: Measurement of abdominal and back muscle strength with and without low back pain. Scand Rehabil Med J 1:60–65, 1969.
65. Nicolaisen T, Jorgensen K: Trunk strength, back muscle endurance and low-back trouble. Scand Rehabil Med J 17:121–127, 1985.
66. Nummi J, et al: Diminished dynamic performance capacity of back and abdominal muscles in concrete reinforcement workers. Scand J Work Environ Health 4:39–46, 1978.
67. Parnianpour M, Nordin M, et al: The triaxial coupling of torque generation of trunk muscles during isometric exertions and the effect of fatiguing isoinertial movements on the motor output and movement patterns. Spine 13:982–992, 1988.
68. Parnianpour M, Li F, et al: A database of isoinertial trunk strength tests against three resistance levels. Spine 14:409–411, 1989.
69. Porter RW, Hibbert C, Wellman P: Backache and the lumbar spinal canal. Spine 5:99–105, 1980.
70. Redfield JT: The low-back x-ray as a pre-employment screening tool in the forest. J Occup Med 13:219–226, 1971.
71. Rothstein JM, Mayhew TP: Clinical uses of isokinetic measurements. Phys Ther 67:1840–1844, 1987.

72. Rowe LM: Low-back pain in industry. J Occup Med 11:161–169, 1969.
73. Rowe ML: Low back disability in industry: Updated position. J Occup Med 13:476–478, 1969.
74. Rowe ML: Backache at Work. Fairport, NY, Perinton Press, 1983.
75. Saal JA, Saal JS: Nonoperative treatment of herniated lumbar intervertebral disc with radiculopathy. Spine 14:431–437, 1989.
76. Seeds RH, et al: Electronic equipment provides accuracy in back injury analysis. Occup Health Saf 1:38–42, 1988.
77. Smidt G, et al: Assessment of abdominal and back extensor function: A quantitative approach and results for chronic low-back patients. Spine 8:211–219, 1983.
78. Smith SS, et al: Quantification of lumbar function. Part I. Isometric and multispeed isokinetic trunk strength measures in sagittal and axial planes in normal subjects. Spine 10:757–764, 1985.
79. Snook SH, Campanelli RA, Hart JW: A study of three preventative approaches to low back injury. J Occup Med 20:478–481, 1978.
80. Snook SH, Jensen RC: Occupational Low Back Pain. New York, Praeger Publishers, 1984.
81. Snook SH: Approaches to the control of back pain in industry: Job design, job placement, and education/training. Spine State Art Rev 2:49–54, 1987.
82. Spengler DM: Back injuries in industry: A retrospective study. Spine 11:241–245, 1986.
83. Thistle HG, et al: Isokinetic contraction: A new concept of resistive exercise. Arch Phys Med Rehabil 48:279–282, 1967.
84. Troup JDG: The perception of back pain and the role of psychophysical tests of lifting capacity. Spine 12:645–657, 1987.
85. Vallfors B: Acute, subacute and chronic LBP: Clinical symptoms, absenteeism, and working environment. Scand J Rehabil Med 11:1–98, 1985.
86. White AA, Gordon SL: Synopsis: Workshop on idiopathic low-back pain. Spine 7:141–149, 1982.
87. Wickstrom G: Effect of work on degenerative back disease: A review. Scand J Work Environ Health 4:1–12, 1978.
88. Wood DJ: Design and evaluation of a back injury program within a geriatric hospital. Spine 12:77–82, 1987.
89. Zeh J, et al: Isometric strength testing: Recommendations based on statistical analysis of the procedure. Spine 11:43–44, 1986.

AVITAL FAST, MD

LOW BACK PAIN IN PREGNANCY: PATHOPHYSIOLOGY, PRESENTATION, TREATMENT

From the Department of
  Rehabilitation Medicine
St. Vincent Hospital and
  Medical Center of New York
New York, New York

Reprint requests to:
Avital Fast, MD
Chairman, Department of
  Rehabilitation Medicine
St. Vincent Hospital and
  Medical Center of New York
153 West 11th Street
New York, NY 10011

It is common knowledge among many obstetricians that a significant number of women develop low back pain (LBP) during pregnancy. In many cases the patients are told that backache may be expected to occur during pregnancy and that the pain will disappear after delivery. Commonly, the patient has severe pain that interferes with her activities of daily living. In spite of the high prevalence of backache during pregnancy, the literature dealing with the subject is not extensive. To this day, in many patients the pathogenesis of LBP during pregnancy remains obscure and a uniform therapeutic approach is still lacking.

EPIDEMIOLOGY AND CLINICAL PRESENTATION

Recent surveys have established that about 50% of pregnant women complain of LBP during pregnancy.[2,8,22] In the majority of these patients the pain does not significantly interfere with daily activities. In about 10% of the patients, however, the pain may be severe, curtail activities, or may force the patient to bed.[2,8] Women with multiple pregnancies tend to be more disabled by the pain than those in their first pregnancy and might be at higher risk of developing sacroiliac joint dysfunction.[8] Patients suffering from occasional backache prior to pregnancy may expect more pain—daily or hourly—during pregnancy. In the majority of the patients the backache may last for a short period of time. In about 6% the painful periods are prolonged and may last more than 6 months.[2]

Many activities may aggravate the pain. The most common involve standing, forward-bending, sitting, lifting, and walking. In about a third of the patients the pain may increase during coughing and sneezing. Many report that lying down or stretching their backs alleviates the pain.[8]

In about 45% of the cases the pain radiates into the lower extremities, mainly the buttocks and thighs. Occasionally the pain may radiate into the leg, but the feet are usually spared.[8,22] In most cases the pain radiates unilaterally. Occasionally it radiates bilaterally.

Pain diagrams clearly demonstrate the aforementioned distribution and are consistent with the patient's complaints.[8] Most women develop LBP between the fifth and seventh months.[8,22] This pattern does not correlate with the distribution of weight gain during pregnancy. If there was a direct correlation between weight gain and LBP during pregnancy, one would expect to see more LBP cases as pregnancy progresses. In effect, however, the number of new LBP cases, beyond seventh month, actually decreases.[8]

Most patients complain of diurnal backache, which is usually attributed to hyperlordosis or fatigue-stress–induced pain. A significant number of patients, however, specifically indicate the occurrence of backache during nighttime.[8,22] In these patients other mechanisms rather than fatigue-stress should be considered, as will be mentioned subsequently.

PATHOGENESIS

A recent survey evaluated the potential contributions of race, weight gain, baby's weight, number of previous pregnancies, number of prior children, age of the mother, and exercise habits to the pathogenesis of LBP during pregnancy.[8] Race was the only variable of statistical significance. Hispanic women had a significantly lower incidence of backache, whereas Caucasian women had a much higher incidence.[8] This surprising ethnic distribution still remains unexplained. Another study has demonstrated that smoking and work requiring lifting and simultaneous turning motions were significantly more common in pregnant women with sacroiliac joint dysfunction and severe low back pain.[2]

At the present state of knowledge, a precise diagnosis of the etiology of LBP during pregnancy still cannot be made in many women. It is felt that the dramatic physiological changes of pregnancy occurring over a short period of time lead to significant alterations in various systems, predisposing the subject to LBP. Some of the changes are visible, e.g., weight gain, whereas others such as hormonal changes are not visible but have extensive influence on maternal physiology.

The average weight gained at term is about 12 kg. During the first trimester there is a very slight weight gain (1.25 kg), whereas during the second and third trimesters, the weight gain in about 5 to 55 kg per trimester. By the ninth month, the body mass is expected to rise by 20%.[5,13] Part of the weight gain is contributed by the dramatic growth of the uterus, which increases from about 30 g to 1400 g. The uterine dimensions increase 150-fold during pregnancy. At term, the uterus with its content contributes an average of 6 kg to maternal weight. The hypertrophied breasts add, on the average, 1–2 kg.[5]

The distending uterus displaces the abdominal wall outward and overstretches the abdominal muscles. This may weaken the muscles and occasionally lead to diastasis recti-separation of the recti muscles. The overstretched abdominal muscles are compromised, resulting in a decreased amount of pressure that can be sustained by the abdominal cavity. This leads to increased stress sustained by the ligaments and bones. The rapidly increasing weight that has to be borne by the unsupported spine puts additional stress on the disc and ligaments, thus exposing them to potential damage. These changes displace the center of gravity upward and forward, rendering it unstable. In order to maintain a stable upright position, the woman has to change her posture and is forced into hyperlordosis. This is combined with anterior tilt of the pelvis. These dramatic and rapidly occurring postural changes forseeably modify the three-dimensional alignment of the lumbar spine and alter the weight distribution of the motion segment. This may consequently lead to reduced biomechanical efficiency of the supporting ligaments and muscles, thereby increasing the stress on static structures, i.e., facet joints.

These mechanical changes during pregnancy may generate local and referred pain.[4] Many authors have emphasized the important role played by the trunk musculature in the pathogenesis of LBP. Suzuki et al. have demonstrated that male patients with LBP had greater fatigability of trunk flexors than control subjects without backache. Fatigability developed more easily in trunk flexors than extensors. Even in patients with short-term LBP, the trunk muscles were significantly weaker. The authors hypothesized that imbalance of strength between flexors and extensors may be a factor contributing to LBP.[30] The relation between decreased muscle strength, endurance, increased fatigability, and backache has been confirmed by others.[19,25] The abdominal muscles play an important role in raising the intra-abdominal pressure by converting the abdominal cavity into a "fluid ball," thus sustaining a significant part of the compressive forces. As a result, the thoracoabdominal cavity actually reduces the stress and the axial compression forces acting on the spine and the discs, in particular.[26]

Recent work established the isometric-isokinetic values for normal trunk muscle strength and endurance in women.[26] Similar studies evaluating these parameters in pregnancy are still lacking.

The effect of pregnancy on abdominal muscle function was recently evaluated by sit-up performance in 164 pregnant women and compared to 164 nonpregnant women.[9] The results demonstrated that in late stages of pregnancy the abdominal muscles become markedly insufficient. The vast majority of women (86.5%) were unable to perform a sit-up in the hook-lying position, whereas 16% could not perform a single sit-up at all. In using this crude method of evaluation, no statistically significant correlation between the ability or inability to perform a sit-up and the existence of backache was found.

Studies utilizing a more scientific quantitative approach, including intraabdominal pressure measurements, may help establish the role played by the compromised abdominal muscles in the pathogenesis of LBP during pregnancy.

The significance of hyperlordosis in the pathogenesis of LBP during pregnancy remains unclear. It is felt that the rapidly changing posture alters the load distribution on the spine, increases the weight borne by the posterior elements, e.g., facets, and predispose to backache. Furthermore, hyperextension of the spine may lead to narrowing of the intervertebral foraminae and the spinal canal and lead to sciatica. Although it is widely accepted that the spine assumes a hyperlordotic posture during pregnancy, to the best of this author's knowledge, no scientific studies have confirmed this. Considering the above, one should remember that the role played by hyperlordosis is far from established and at times is portrayed as irrelevant.[11,12]

Many gynecologists are of the opinion that the pelvis and, in particular, the sacroiliac joints play a key role in the pathogenesis of LBP and referred pain during pregnancy. In this context, a review of some of the important hormonal changes that occur during pregnancy, specifically those related to relaxin, is appropriate.

In spite of the fact that the hormone relaxin has been identified and its structure has been characterized, its physiological significance is not yet fully established. Relaxin is secreted from the corpus luteum. It reaches its peak activity during the first trimester. Concentrations in the third trimester are lower than those found in early and mid-pregnancy.[20] Relaxin affects fibroblasts in various structures, especially in pelvic joints. Relaxation of these joints occurs in normal pregnancy and is an essential process that enables the pelvis to accommodate the fetus during late stages of pregnancy and delivery. Comparative symphyseal measurements, via x-ray studies, of nonpregnant nulliparae and pregnant primiparae have clearly demonstrated the significant separation of the pubis symphysis during pregnancy. These changes were already established by the end of the fifth month, at which time there was no direct pressure by the fetus. Physical examination further demonstrated excessive pubic motility.[1] Since the pelvis is constructed in the form of a ring, displacement in one joint—the pubis—has to lead to corresponding changes in the sacroiliac joints, leading to sacroiliac instability and strain. These changes render the pelvis unstable and interfere with its capacity to handle static and dynamic stresses, which may become excessive during pregnancy and as a result LBP may occur. Sacroiliac joint problems may present clinically with backache, pain over the buttocks, and tenderness over the pubis, or pain radiating over the lateral aspects of the buttock and anterolateral aspect of the thigh. Many pregnant patients display precisely these symptoms.[1]

An important study associating relaxin and pelvic pain was recently published by MacLennan et al.[21] They measured the serum relaxin levels in 35 pregnant patients who complained of severe pelvic pain and pelvic joint instability. Included in this group of patients were only those who were severely disabled and in whom clinical examination and testing confirmed the diagnosis. Many of these patients had to be hospitalized because of their inability to ambulate. Serum relaxin samples from asymptomatic pregnant subjects were obtained for comparison. The study documented a highly statistically significant increase in serum relaxin levels in the symptomatic group. Furthermore, the highest relaxin levels were found in those patients who were the most incapacitated.[21]

A prospective study of 862 pregnant women found that about 9% of them develop severe pain that interferes with activities of daily living. In two-thirds of these patients, physical examination, including provocative tests, detected sacroiliac joint dysfunction. Symphysiolysis was also significantly more common among those with sacroiliac joint dysfunction than among pregnant women without backache. Many women with sacroiliac joint dysfunction complained of significant pain emanating from the pubic area.[2] Indeed, softening of the symphysis pubis may be an important factor leading to increased stress upon the sacroiliac joints and thus may contribute to sacroiliac joint dysfunction.[7]

Pubic bone instability can be diagnosed by crepitus and tenderness over the area, with an associated gaping pubic defect.[31] During alternate leg standing, the unstable pubic bones can be felt to move. This may actually be documented, after delivery, by x-ray studies performed during alternate leg standing.[16]

In sacroiliac joint dysfunction, even in the presence of pain radiating down into the buttock or thigh, the neurological examination remains normal and no tension signs should be found.

During pregnancy, the intervertebral discs are subjected to increased mechanical stresses that may result in disc herniation. The increased stress is brought about by carrying additional weight, abdominal muscle insufficiency, and ligamentous laxity, particularly of the posterior longitudinal ligament. The increased pressures and stresses incurred during normal delivery may further jeopardize a patient with a protruded disc. These facts support the view that pregnancy predisposes to the development of herniated discs.[27]

In an extensive epidemiological study, Kelsey et al. concluded that pregnancies that terminate with live births increase the risk of herniated lumbar discs. Furthermore, the risk increases with subsequent births. Women with L5 herniated discs averaged 3.09 live births compared to 1.91 live births in their controls.[14]

It is, therefore, not surprising that herniated discs occur during pregnancy. What is surprising is that the number of reported herniated discs during pregnancy is very low.

In a review of 48,760 consecutive deliveries, only five pregnant patients with symptoms and signs of herniated lumbosacral discs were identified, an incidence of 1:10,000. The pain was initially limited to the back. Radicular pain sciatica was more common toward the end of pregnancy. In each case, the straight leg raising test was markedly limited. In two patients a foot drop was documented. Nerve conduction studies were uniformly normal. Electromyography detected denervation in a radicular distribution, including the paraspinal muscles. All the patients were initially managed by bed rest, pelvic traction, thermotherapy, and TENS. A Cesarian section was performed towards the end of pregnancy. Post-delivery myelograms demonstrated large herniated discs.[17] Only a few magnetic resonance imaging studies, performed during pregnancy, have been published thus far. These studies yield conflicting results. In some, an increased incidence of disc herniation during pregnancy, particularly at the L5–S1 level, is reported.[23,24] Other researchers do not find any difference in the prevalence of lumbar disc degeneration and disc bulging in pregnant and nonpregnant control groups.[28] At present, magnetic resonance imaging studies are not considered safe during pregnancy and are not routinely done. Whenever safe imaging studies are introduced, more information concerning the spine and discs during pregnancy will become available.

Maternal lumbosacral plexus paralysis, a well-described syndrome that can mimic a herniated disc, can occur in small women bearing large babies. As the baby's head descends into the pelvis, just prior to or during delivery, it may compress nerve trunks in the pelvis. As the lumbosacral trunk, the superior gluteal nerve, or the obturator nerve course downward over the pelvic bony brim, they become susceptible.

In spite of superficial clinical similarities, certain features help differentiate between the two conditions. Herniated discs may occur throughout pregnancy. Lumbosacral plexus paralysis usually occurs following prolonged and difficult deliveries. Whereas the prognosis of herniated discs is usually favorable, plexus paralysis often results in prolonged or lasting disability. In the former, lumbar pain, spasm, and stiffness are common. Plexus lesions, however, do not affect the back. In herniated discs, pain is the predominant symptom and is usually not accompanied by frank neurological symptoms. Plexus lesions frequently present as foot drop.[15]

A significant number of pregnant women (up to 35%) specifically complain of night backache.[8,22] At times the pain is severe enough to disturb sleep and forces the patient out of bed.[10]

The factors contributing to LBP during daytime activities, i.e., hyperlordosis, musculoskeletal fatigue, and excessive movement of pelvic joints, do not seem to play a major role during sleep. The exact pathophysiological processes that lead to night backache are not yet established.

It has been shown that during pregnancy the uterus may obstruct or completely occlude the inferior vena cava. This may occur in the supine and also in side-lying positions.[18] During the night there is redistribution of fluids from the extracellular space into the vascular system. The ensuing hypervolemia, combined with obstruction of the inferior vena cava, may increase the pressure in the pelvic veins and structures subserved by them, e.g., vertebral bodies. The veins and vessels inside the vertebral bodies are supplied by a plexus of unmyelinated fibers. These nerve fibers constitute a vascular pain receptor system. It is hypothesized that in women with inadequate collateral circulation, excessive pressure may gradually build up during the night. The excessive pressure, combined with increased progesterone-mediated venous distensibility, leads to vascular overdistension.

Persistent venous stasis may then cause stagnation hypoxemia and local metabolic disturbances that affect the neural structures. The combined impact of these mechanisms may lead to the development of night backache during pregnancy.[10]

MANAGEMENT

The chances of a successful therapeutic regimen increase when a clear, precise diagnosis can be established. In many LBP cases, including LBP during pregnancy, the clinician does not have a "tissue diagnosis"—that is, a clear understanding of the pathogenesis of pain. In these cases, a trial and error approach is utilized, i.e., flexion versus extension exercises. In a pregnant patient presenting with severe LBP, every effort to rule out pathological processes that may jeopardize the mother or the fetus should be made. Since radiological studies cannot be routinely performed during pregnancy, the physician has to rely on the history and physical examination. A detailed neurological examination is of extreme importance. In selected cases, electrodiagnostic studies should be obtained to help establish the diagnosis and a proper therapeutic course. In the presence of long-tract sings or evidence of myelopathy, imaging studies including MRI and even myelography may be indicated. The literature dealing with management of backache during pregnancy is scarce. In many papers anecdotal and personal experiences are cited. Prospective, comparative studies dealing with this entity are scant.

In the majority of cases the most common cause of LBP during pregnancy is pelvic instability combined with modified body mechanics. Treatment in these cases should be based on the following guidelines: rest, exercises, and support. Many pregnant women very quickly learn that in order to get through the day, several rest periods are required.

The women should be advised to refrain from activities that increase pain and to adopt positions that bring about pain relief. Avoiding prolonged standing, a position that entails hyperlordosis and anterior pelvic tilt, is advised. Guidance regarding faulty postures and proper body mechanics should be given. Prenatal classes combining lectures and exercises are the best educational medium. The exercises should include mild low-impact aerobics, exercises specifically tailored to tone and strengthen the pelvic floor musculature, pelvic tilt exercises, stretching exercises, and relaxation techniques.

Whenever the pain persists and is severe enough to compromise function, the patient should be advised to stop working and stay off her feet. A trochanteric belt or a supporting abdominal girdle can be of significant help in the late months of pregnancy.

Cady et al., in a prospective study on fire fighters, have shown that fit individuals tend to develop fewer back problems than non-fit individuals.[3] Fast et al. have demonstrated that nonpregnant women who spend more than 4 hours per week on physical fitness had less backache than women who exercised 1–4 hours per week. The difference between the two groups reached a statistically significant level. In pregnant women, however, this trend was not present.[9] Studies evaluating the effect of high fitness prior to pregnancy on LBP are still missing. It is advisable to recommend to a woman who suffers from significant LBP during pregnancy that she increase her fitness level prior to the next pregnancy and maintain a moderate level of activity during pregnancy.

Many therapeutic modalities such as ultrasound, short wave diathermy, and microwave are considered unsafe during pregnancy. Others, i.e., massage, superficial moist heat, or cooling, can be used. The latter modalities combined with stretching exercises may be very helpful in patients with muscle spasms. Mobilization and manipulation are occasionally performed during pregnancy.[2,6] Their efficacy and long-term effects have not been yet established. Transcutaneous electrical nerve stimulation (TENS) has gained popularity in the management of labor pain. However, it has not yet been approved as a safe modality in the treatment of backache during pregnancy. In patients with herniated discs that compromise the nerve roots, close monitoring by frequent neurological examination is called for. In the case of progressive unrelenting neurological deterioration, or in the presence of cauda equina syndrome, immediate surgical intervention should be considered.[29]

I hope that future research dealing with backache and sciatica during pregnancy will enable us to adopt more scientifically proven methods and develop specific guidelines for management of LBP during pregnancy.

REFERENCES

1. Abramson D, Roberts S, Wilson P: Relaxation of the pelvic joints in pregnancy. Surg Gynecol Obstet 58:595–613, 1934.
2. Berg G, Hammar M, Moller-Nielsen J, et al: Low back pain during pregnancy. Obstet Gynecol 71:71–75, 1988.
3. Cady L, Bischoff P, O'Connell E, et al: Strength and fitness and subsequent back injuries in fire fighters. J Occup Med 21:269–272, 1979.
4. Cherry S, Berkowitz R, Kase N: Medical, Surgical and Gynecologic Complications of Pregnancy. Baltimore, Wilkins & Wilkins, 1985.
5. Chesley L: Weight changes and water balance in normal and toxic pregnancy. Am J Obstet Gynecol 48:565–593, 1944.
6. Epstein J, Benton J, Browder J, et al: Treatment of low back pain and sciatic syndromes during pregnancy. NY State J Med 59:1757–1768, 1959.
7. Farbrot E: The relationship of the effect and pain of pregnancy to the anatomy of the pelvis. Acta Radiol 38:403–419, 1952.

8. Fast A, Shapiro D, Ducommun E, et al: Low back pain in pregnancy. Spine 12:368–371, 1987.

9. Fast A, Weiss L, Ducommun E, et al: Low back pain in pregnancy: Abdominal muscles sit-up performance and back pain. Spine 15:28–30, 1990.

10. Fast A, Weiss L, Parikh S, Hertz G: Night backache in pregnancy: Hypothetical pathophysiological mechanisms. Am J Phys Med Rehabil 68:227–229, 1989.

11. Frymoyer J: Back pain and sciatica. N Engl J Med 318:291–300, 1988.

12. Hansson T, Bigos S, Beecher P, Wortley M: The lumbar lordosis in acute and chronic low back pain. Spine 10:154–155, 1985.

13. Jacobson H: Diet in pregnancy. N Engl J Med 297:1051–1053, 1977.

14. Kelsey J, Greenberg R, Hardy R, Johnson M: Pregnancy and the syndrome of herniated lumbar intervertebral disc: An epidemiological study. Yale J Biol Med 48:361–365, 1975.

15. King A: Neurologic conditions occurring as complications of pregnancy. Arch Neurol Psychiatry 63:611–644, 1950.

16. Laban M, Meerschaert J, Taylor R, Tabor H: Symphyseal and sacroiliac joint pain and associated with pubic symphysis instability. Arch Phys Med Rehabil 59:470–472, 1978.

17. Laban M, Perrin J, Latimer F: Pregnancy and the herniated lumbar disc. Arch Phys Med Rehabil 64:319–321, 1983.

18. Lees M, Scott D, Kerr M, Taylor S: The circulatory effects of recumbent postural change in late pregnancy. Clin Sci 32:453–465, 1967.

19. Leino P, Aro S, Hasan J: Trunk muscle function and low back disorders: A ten year follow-up study. J Chron Dis 40:289–296, 1987.

20. MacLennan A, Nicolson R, Green R: Serum relaxin in pregnancy. Lancet 2:241–243, 1986.

21. MacLennan A, Nicolson R, Green R, Bath M: Serum relaxin and pelvic pain of pregnancy. Lancet 2:243–245, 1986.

22. Mantle M, Greenwood R, Currey H: Backache in pregnancy. Rheumatol Rehabil 16:95–101, 1977.

23. McCarthy S: Magnetic resonance imaging in obstetrics and gynecology. Magn Reson Imaging 4:59–66, 1986.

24. McCarthy S, Stark D, Filly R, et al: Obstetrical magnetic resonance imaging: Maternal anatomy. Radiology 154:427–432, 1985.

25. McNeill T, Warwick D, Andersson G, Schultz A: Trunk strengths in attempted flexion, extension and lateral bending in healthy subjects and patients with low-back disorders. Spine 5:529–537, 1980.

26. Nordin M, Kahanovitz N, Verderame R, et al: Normal trunk muscle strength and endurance in women and the effect of exercises and electrical stimulation. Part I: Normal endurance and trunk muscle strength in 101 women. Spine 12:105–111, 1987.

27. O'Connell J: Lumbar disc protrusions in pregnancy. J Neurol Neurosurg Psychiatry 23:138–141, 1960.

28. Powell M, Wilson M, Szypryt P, et al: Prevalence of lumbar disc degeneration observed by magnetic resonance in symptomless women. Lancet 2:1366–1367, 1986.

29. Sands R: Backache of pregnancy. A method of treatment. Obstet Gynecol 12:670–676, 1958.

30. Suzuki N, Endo S: A quantitative study of trunk muscle strength and fatigability in the low-back-pain syndrome. Spine 8:69–74, 1983.

31. Taylor R, Sonson R: Separation of the pubic symphysis. An underrecognized peripartum complication. J Reprod Med 3:203–206, 1986.

MYRON M. LaBAN, MD, FACP

"WHIPLASH": ITS EVALUATION AND TREATMENT

From the Department of Physical
  Medicine and Rehabilitation
William Beaumont Hospital
Royal Oak, Michigan

Reprint requests to:
Myron M. LaBan, MD, FACP
Director, Department of Physical
  Medicine and Rehabilitation
William Beaumont Hospital
Royal Oak, MI 48072

The generic "whiplash" injury affecting the cervical spine occurs most often as a result of violent hyperextension of the head on the shoulders when one vehicle is struck from behind by another. Osseous as well as articular, ligamentous, and other soft tissue injuries may occur, culminating in prolonged disability with the potential for subsequent litigation. The range of severity of residual neck injury depends on multiple factors related to the accelerative forces incurred and the relative movement of the head on the trunk. A spectrum of injury, ranging from fracture/dislocation of the cervical spine associated with variable degrees of residual quadriplegia to injuries causing death. Motor vehicle accidents in the United States are responsible for approximately half of the traumatic deaths. Over 75% of these fatalities occur in automobiles, trucks, or on motorcycles. Of the remainder, 20% are pedestrians, an additional 2% are bicyclists, and 2% are associated with train collisions. Six thousand passenger car occupants die each year. Death in this group is most often related to spinal cord damage secondary to neck dislocation or fracture. One-third of these victims are ejected from their vehicle. Ten percent of those with a cervical spinal cord injury survive. Thirty percent of these (Fig. 1) are left with a persistent pattern of incomplete quadriplegia.[1,11,31] The recent adoption of national set belt has helped to improve this record.[50]

Fortunately, of the estimated 3,800,000 rear-end collisions that occur annually in the U.S., relatively few result in death or quadriplegias.

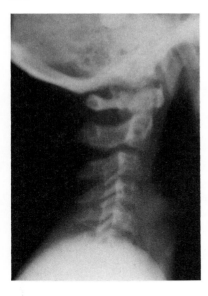

FIGURE 1. Teenager with fracture-dislocation C2 on C3 with quadriparesis.

Instead, the vast majority are associated with only residual complaints of neck and shoulder pain secondary to soft tissue injury without objective neural or osseous spinal dyscrasia. Acceleration-hyperextension injuries to the cervical spine continue to remain as challenging a problem of medical management as they were in 1867, when they were primarily associated with railroad accidents.[9] Then as now, the term "whiplash" (coined in 1928 by Crowe[46]) all too often projects a negative image of a guileful patient wearing a cervical collar, sustained on one side by plaintiff's attorney and on the other by a compliant physician. The patient who initially presented with complaints of pain has become the "painful patient." In this process he has become addicted to the pain, real or imagined, for the many secondary gain "benefits," including, among others, attention and financial reward. Unfortunately, our liability system of reimbursement has both the potential and capacity to corrupt all of the concerned parties, including the accident victim as well as both the plaintiff and defense attorneys. In this scenario the treating physician often discovers that his initial observations and therapeutic ministrations are unimportant in the process. Six months later the "independent" medical examiner finds "nothing wrong" on behalf of his insurance company employer.

The litigious process itself becomes the preoccupying focus of all of the concerned parties. The patient's complaints and the corresponding clinical findings are expediently ignored! In this regard, clinical experience would suggest that even in a disparate patient population given the same pathomechanics of neck injury, the commonality of brachiocephalic complaints would suggest similar pathophysiology. Contrary to the popular misconception, persistent symptoms associated with cervical hyperextension injuries are in fact real! The subsequent disabilities may all too often prove to be refractive to treatment.

Shortly after an auto accident, complaints of neck pain can occur in up to 30% of car occupants. In over half of these cases the onset of symptoms may be delayed for 24 hours.[54] In the long term, another 30% will also report symptoms of cervical pain. Rear impacts produce neck injuries twice as often as frontal impacts. Front-seat occupants have a 30% greater likelihood of incurring a neck injury than those in the rear seat. The driver is at slightly less risk than the front-seat passenger, probably due to the immediate bracing effect of the steering wheel. Age itself appears to be an unrelated factor, with women and taller passengers more vulnerable to neck injury. The presence of antecedent degenerative changes of the cervical spine appears to predispose the patient to persistent symptoms.[4]

Injury to the neck following acceleration/deceleration injuries is most often clinically significant when the head is hyperextended on the shoulders. In this circumstance there are relatively few impediments to cervical spine hyperextension short of the occiput striking the posterior chest wall. Relative to the normal range of cervical forward and lateral flexion, hyperextension may far exceed anatomical and physiological restraints that normally limit movement. Variable degrees of neck rotation significantly reduce cervical spine flexibility and extension at the zygoapophyseal joints. At 45 degrees of cervical rotation, physiological extension is decreased by one-half. Macnab, in his review of 575 patients with "whiplash syndrome," noted that those with persistent symptoms had a history of a significant cervical hyperextension injury.[45] In this same series, out of a selected group of patients involved in litigation, 45% remained symptomatic 2 or more years after settlement. Although this would appear to be an excessively large number of patients with residual complaints, most large patient series would confirm that up to 15% of patients remain significantly symptomatic and require on-going medical treatment.[21] In another series, 26% of patients continued to have intermittent neck pain 1 year after injury and 4% had continuous discomfort.[14] Juhl and Seerup reported that 30% of their neck injured patients lost work time,[29] while Larder noted that 59% of his patients reported some disruption in their daily routines many months after the accidents, particularly during work and driving activities.[42]

BIOMECHANICS OF INJURY

Injury to the cervical spine in motor vehicle crashes occurs as a result of the brief but immense decelerative forces that are associated with the collision. Within 0.20 seconds of a crash, the occupants decelerate to zero speed. The forces of gravity experienced by the operator vary directly as the square of the speed and inversely to the stopping distance: $g = (mph)^2 / (30 \times stopping distance [ft])$.[62] When the vehicle is at rest and is struck from behind, the sudden acceleration of the stationary car and its occupants can hyperextend the relatively heavy head (5 kg) on the shoulders. The sudden posterior displacement of the head not only loads the cervical zygoapophyseal joints but may also violently stretch the anterior cervical compartment tissues and simultaneously hyperextend the torso on the pelvis. Rebound cervical flexion may also occur, particularly if the impacted vehicle is thrust forward into another car. This moment may be amplified by a reflex-modulated contraction of the neck flexors reacting to the initial cervical spinal hyperextension.[26]

At speeds of less then 15 mph a forewarned driver may escape significant injury by bracing himself against the steering wheel. When the impact exceeds 20 mph, the unrestrained driver may find himself in nearly a horizontal position as the seat back breaks with the neck subjected to axial distractive forces rather than those of extension.[44] Properly positioned head restraints as well as seat belts together can act to maintain safe positioning of the passengers. However, the use of seat belts alone without the added protection of a head rest may, by restraining forward motion of the trunk, amplify neck excursion in extension. Neck restraints have reduced the incidence of cervical spine injury following rear impacts by 17%. In Great Britain there was an immediate 25% reduction in death and serious injuries to car occupants following implementation of mandatory seat belts in 1983. Unfortunately, at the same time there was a concomitant increase in the incidence of neck soft tissue injuries.[48]

Additionally, specific patterns of injury have been sporadically reported in association with the use of various restraints,[55] including fractures of the lumbar vertebral bodies (Chance),[18] visceral injuries, myocardial contusions,[23] placental hematomas in pregnancy,[17] and sternal[16] and clavicular fractures (Fig. 2), as well as breast injuries.[13]

PATHOLOGIC CONSEQUENCES OF INJURY

Research on both human cadavers and primates using both staged auto crashes and sled testing have demonstrated reproducible patterns of extension injury to the neck. Depending on the force of injury, variable degrees of muscle strain were produced, ranging from minor tears of the sternocleidomastoid and longus colli muscles to severe tearing of these muscles in association with retropharyngeal hematoma formation. Additional hemorrhages were also identified with the esophagus and between the seven intermuscular fascial planes of the neck. On occasion, associated damage to the cervical sympathetic plexus may be seen. When significant damage occurred to the ventral muscles of the neck, disruption of the anterior longitudinal ligament of the spine with disc separation from the adjacent vertebrae could be identified. Macnab, in monkey studies, noted that even several months after disc injury roentgenographic studies

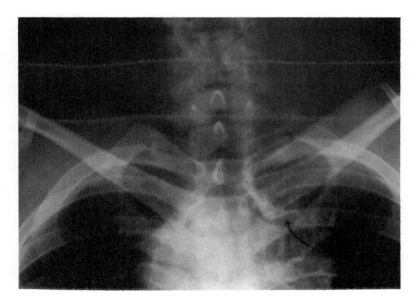

FIGURE 2.   Right sternoclavicular joint subluxation secondary to shoulder strap trauma.

failed to identify the disc disorder.[44] Cadaver experiments have confirmed these impressions, with intervertebral disc damage being a frequent finding at autopsy. These disruptions occur most frequently at levels most affected by osteochondrotic change. Hemorrhages have also been observed around nerve roots and in the adventitia of the vertebral arteries.[8,30] These autopsy findings, although obtained in carefully structured but artificial circumstances, do suggest that, given significant trauma, well-defined anatomical lesions can occur. Clearly, these observations have valid clinical significance relative to the evaluation and treatment of whiplash injury.

CLINICAL SYNDROMES

The vast majority of cervical injuries, up to 98%, are low grade. In these circumstances sudden hyperextension of the neck can stretch the longus colli and scaleni muscles as well as the pretracheal fascia. Often this is associated with actual or perceived swelling of the sternocleidomastoid muscles. Neck stiffness associated with occipital headache is a common associated complaint. This full symptom complex may not manifest itself until 24 hours after injury.

Pre-existing cervical spondylosis can predispose to persistent cervical radicular complaints, with symptoms of paresthesia in the dermatomal distribution of the root (i.e., thumb (C6), middle finger (C7), and ring and little fingers [C8–T1]). Similarly, myotome pain radiation in the root distribution to distal muscles includes C5–C6 to the proximal shoulder muscle groups, C7 to the triceps and pectoralis major, and C8–T1 to the distal hand intrinsics. Ligamentous or articular referred pain from the zygoapophyseal joints can also be referred in a sclerotome distribution, with articular C5–C6 pain to the upper shoulder, C6–C7 to the medial scapular border, and C8–T1 to the inferior medial scapular border. Likewise, headaches in the distribution of occipital nerves can be associated with spondyloarthritic changes of the upper cervical vertebrae. Symptoms often fluctuate in severity and can reoccur even with minor degrees of physical activity.[47,51]

Injuries of greater severity to the neck (2–3%) are usually associated with significant property damage. Again, injury to the pretracheal areas can produce tearing of the longus colli and scaleni as well as the sternocleidomastoid muscles. The resultant swelling may make it impossible to button a shirt collar. Hoarseness as well as dysphasia may also occur secondary to stretching of the recurrent laryngeal nerves and the esophagus.[25] Vertigo, tinnitus, nausea, and facial dysesthesia can be associated with irritation of the sympathetic nerve trunks in juxtaposition to the carotid and vertebral arteries. Visual aberrations are a common complaint, with symptoms either of blurring or difficulty in focusing. Periorbital ecchymosis and/or Horner's syndrome may also be identified.[3,24]

Symptoms are usually severe in these instances and begin immediately after the accident with brachiocephalic complaints intensifying for 2 to 3 days post-injury. Concomitant mobility of the neck is often markedly restricted, with severe headache radiating to both the occiput as well as to the temples.[2] Cervical radicular signs and symptoms are usually more evident with identifiable reflex changes, myotome weakness, and occasional muscular atrophy. With increasing violence of neck trauma, significant and often irreparable damage can occur to the spine itself, the cervical cord, and the brain. Unrestrained acute neck hyperextension can rupture the anterior longitudinal ligament and the anterior annulus of the disc, producing both nerve root and cord damage.[7] Even without fracture/dislocation of the cervical vertebrae, quadriplegia can be induced by pre-existing spondyloarthritis or cervical spinal canal stenosis.[56] Distraction of the vertebral arteries can produce posterior fossa neurologic symptoms ranging from vertigo and ataxia to occipital lobe and brain stem ischemia or infarction.[53] Closed head injury can also occur and is associated in these circumstances with the shearing effect of brain acceleration within the closed confines of the bony skull.[20]

EVALUATION AND TREATMENT

Individually and together, the multivariant syndromes associated with cervical hyperextension injury can present with a confusing mélange of complaints. Appropriate treatment in this regard is predicated on identifying the primary disorder and expeditiously treating it. Among those commonly recognized in the pathogenesis of post-traumatic neck pain are occipital neuralgia, temporomandibular joint arthropathy, cervical vertigo, and radiculopathy, as well as myofascial and thoracic outlet syndromes. Brachiocephalic syndromes precipitating reduced shoulder mobility can be compounded by developing bicepital tendonitis, subdeltoid bursitis, and ultimately a shoulder periarthrosis.

Occipital Neuralgia

Symptoms of occipital neuralgia include point tenderness over the occipital notch where the greater occipital nerve penetrates the semispinalis and trapezius muscles at their insertion on the occiput. Unlike other spinal nerves, the ganglia of the C2 spinal roots lie exposed on the vertebral arch of the axis. In this position they are vulnerable to crushing between the bony arches of the atlas and axis during forced hyperextension of the head. Additional complaints include severe headache in the retro-orbital, temporal, and parietal, as well as occipital, areas, scalp "cramps," and burning dysesthesias, which may be described by patients as "my hair is on fire." Occipital neuralgia has been ascribed to over 200 causes including post-traumatic lesions of the cervical cranial junctions and unilateral cervical degenerative arthrosis of the C1–C2 articulations with C2 nerve root involvement.[27] The diagnosis of occipital neuralgia can be substantiated by increased discomfort from direct digital pressure over the symptomatic occipital notch. Arthrosis of the C1–C2 vertebrae can best be recognized on an anteroposterior roentgenographic view of the odontoid process or by CT scan.

Patients who do not respond to physical therapy, including ultrasound following ice massage and intermittent cervical traction, often do well with the simple expedient of local injection of steroid and Xylocaine in the area of the occipital notch. Relief of symptoms in this regard has the dual benefit of being therapeutic and simultaneously confirming the clinical diagnosis.[15]

Arthropathies of the Temporomandibular Joint

Internal derangement of the temporomandibular joints can occur with cervical hyperextension injuries.[52] Complaints of localized pain in addition to associated headache in the occipital, retro-orbital, temporal, and parietal areas are not uncommon. Diagnostic signs include limited mouth opening and reduced lateral jaw movement, as well as painful crepitis or "clicking" of the involved articulation. Palpation of the temporalis muscle above the zygomatic arch with teeth clenched may demonstrate reduced effort on the symptomatic side. If frank articular dislocation can be identified, it can be manually reduced. Additional treatment may include a mandibular repositioning device as well as a night-bite splint.[19]

Cervical Vertigo

Following cervical hyperextension injuries, many patients complain of positional vertigo often associated with occipital as well as fascial sensory aberrations, ranging from a loss of sensation to severe burning pain complaints.[57] The disturbances in equilibrium first noted by Magnus in 1924 are described by patients as "falling in space" or the perception on turning and stopping as a continuance or "sliding" motion. The studies of Barré and Lieou postulated that irritation of the cervical sympathetic nerves produce circulatory disorders of either the vertebral or the internal auditory arteries supplying the vestibular centers causing cervical vertigo.[244] Other investigators have also noted a close association between neck pain following whiplash injuries and vertigo. Although, all researchers agree that the dysequilibrium is most probably due to a dysfunction of afferent nerve fibers to the vestibular nuclei, there are remaining questions as to which anatomical structures initiate these impulses. In one report, "hypertonicity" of the cervical muscle has been suggested. Primary trauma to the cervical zygoapophyseal joints, particularly when cervical arthrosis is present, may also be another. An interplay between the primative "righting reflex" of the neck and the cervical zygoapophyseal joints biased by injury to these articulations may give rise to falsely modulated afferent input to the vestibular nuclei. Inaccurate accommodation at any one moment to spatial changes related to head and trunk positioning may give rise to cervical vertigo.

Facial dysesthesias with complaints of numbness or increased pain can also be attributed to a traumatic neuropathy of the upper cervical roots. The descending tract of the fifth cranial nerve carries with it associated fibers of cranial nerves V, VII, IX and X descending to the level of the upper cervical roots. The axons within this tract carry impulses of pain, temperature, and gross tactile stimulation of the face, the ear, and the scalp as high as the vertex of the skull. At cervical levels C3–C4 these axons cross the spinal cord and provide afferent fibers to form the ascending sensory path, the ventral secondary ascending tract of V. At their most caudal level they are positioned to interact with the upper cervical roots.[49]

Intermittent cervical traction therapy following thermotherapy can be successfully employed in dealing with the triad of symptoms related to occipital neuralgia, facial dysesthesia, and cervical vertigo. These modalities effectively and efficiently treat both a traumatic neuropathy of the second cervical spinal nerve as well as the associated arthropathy of the cervical articulations.[12]

Cervical Radiculopathy

Persistent radicular complaints following cervical hyperextension injuries may also require treatment. Symptoms are often highly variable, from those of a "numb thumb" in the dermatone distribution of C6 root to those of low-grade discomfort along the inferior medial scapular border in the sclerotome distribution of the C8–T1 roots. A post-traumatic C7 radiculopathy can present as severe anterior chest pain in its myotome distribution to the pectoralis major. The immediate concern of the male patient (Fig. 3) may be an impending "heart attack" and, in the female, "breast pain" associated with a suspected malignancy. Confusion in this regard may delay appropriate diagnosis and treatment.[40] The evaluation of a cervical radiculopathy is based on the demonstration both of the presence of a positive ipsilateral cervical foraminal closure test (Spurling's sign) and co-existent weakness in the myotome of the symptomatic root on manual muscle testing. Other useful examinations in diagnosis include the manual cervical

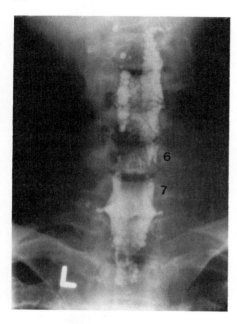

FIGURE 3. Forty-nine year old male with cervical hyperextension injury. Cervical spondyloarthropathy clinically masking a C6–C7 herniated disc presenting as acute chest pain.

distraction and the shoulder abduction tests, which respectively reduce both nerve root compression and tension.[5]

Manual muscle testing can be utilized by employing the "break" maneuver, whereby the patient is given a maximal advantage of position and strength. The examiner subsequently "breaks" the involved muscle, comparing one side to the other. This is the most useful technique in assessing the presence of a cervical root syndrome. A smooth, asymmetric "give" in both the triceps (radial nerve C7–C8) and the pronator teres (median nerve C6–C7) would suggest compromise of the common C7 root.[37]

Electromyographic studies are useful in corroborating the presence and severity of cervical root lesions. However, two caveats must be acknowledged! Unfortunately, acute EMG findings lag 2 weeks behind the patient's actual clinical state. But, after an initial 3-day delay, the immediate status of motor unit innervation and nerve conduction velocity can be followed in real time. In the second instance, EMG is a test of motor dysfunction. If the sensory root is solely compromised and the motor root spared, the EMG examination may be normal. This is often the case with cervical radiculopathies. At cervical spine levels, in approximately 50% of instances there is a separation of the motor and sensory roots at the neural foraminal levels. This discrete separation of the dorsal and ventral fibers enhances the opportunity for motor sparing, even in the presence of severe sensory symptoms. Conversely, motor compromise only can occur as well, without sensory complaint.[40]

Cervical spinal evoked potentials (SEPs) are useful in evaluating the presence of cervical spine myelopathies (Fig. 4). An asymmetric or slowed response to distal upper and lower extremity stimulation may be diagnostic, suggesting the presence of a cervical spine stenosis. However, in the presence of a cervical myelopathy above the C6 level, upper extremity stimulation responses

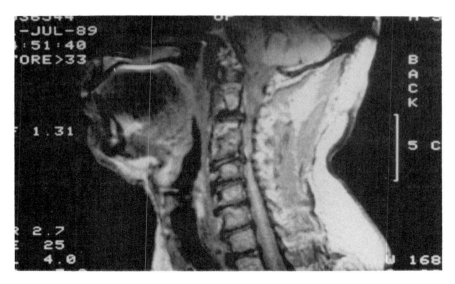

FIGURE 4.   Sixty-five year old male with cervical hyperextension injury. Transient Babinski's associated with MRI and SSEP evidence of spinal stenosis and cervical myelopathy.

are less often abnormal than those performed in the lower extremity. In a suspected myelopathy where overt physical signs are minimal, the SEPs appear to be more sensitive than the clinical examination.[36]

Treatment

The treatment of post-traumatic neck pain is empiric. Initially, analgesics including nonsteroidal anti-inflammatory drugs are effective. As a group, muscle relaxants are soporifics. If putting the patient to sleep is the desired effect, they may be appropriate. Cervical collars and/or braces are initially useful for restricting neck motion. The Thomas soft collar obviously provides less support than a custom-molded plastic orthosis that restrains movement by 50 to 70% but is also more expensive and less comfortable. After an initial week of recovery, the patient should be weaned from these supports as soon as possible before they become psychologic "badges of disability."

Thermotherapy using either superficial heat and/or deep diathermy (i.e., ultrasound) in most instances provides excellent analgesia. In addition, cold, including ice packs or ice massage, can also be effective in treatment. Usually in the more acute stage, ice treatment provides the most significant analgesia. Later, heat is more effective and serves as an excellent precursor to other treatment. Early in treatment, exercise should be encouraged to retain or regain cervical flexibility. Later, a strengthening program should be introduced that includes both active isometric and isotonic exercises.[43]

Intermittent cervical traction with the neck in 30 degrees of flexion, initiated at 15 pounds and then increased to 30 pounds over time, is effective in treating cervical radiculopathy.[10] The reclining and sitting positions are equally therapeutic. Continuous in-bed, low-weight (5-pound) cervical traction, aside from the enforced bed rest, is relatively ineffective. A clinical trial of manual cervical

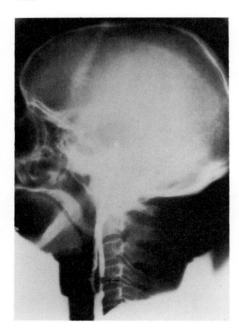

FIGURE 5. Post-traumatic cervical radiculopathy associated with a right carotid bruit. Arteriography demonstrates a carotid lumen of less than 1 mm in a 58-year-old male.

distraction is a useful diagnostic maneuver that can predict a successful response to mechanical intermittent cervical traction therapy. Following an automobile accident and prior to treatment with cervical traction, every patient should have cervical spine x-rays to exclude fractures and/or dislocations. They should also be clinically examined both for signs of myelopathy[38] and the presence of carotid bruits (Fig. 5) as a harbinger of carotid artery stenosis.[39] When associated temporomandibular joint complaints are also present, either padding the jaws or the use of an occipital strap suspension can be recommended.

Traction can actually increase pain complaints when initiated too early or when either a concurrent myofascial and/or thoracic outlet syndrome is present. Attempting cervical traction during the acute phase is often counterproductive. In this phase of recovery, rest rather than active therapy, with the exception of thermotherapy, is recommended. During the acute and chronic phases of neck pain following cervical hyperextension injuries, the myofascial syndromes may become the preeminent source of continuing symptoms.[32] Stretching the painful muscle acutely often increases discomfort. Isolated myofascial nodules and palpable masses within the trapezius, as well as other "trigger points," can reproduce well-recognized patterns of pain referral. These painful sites can be successfully treated singularly or in combination with ice massage, vasocoolant sprays, ultrasound, cervical mobilization exercises, deep-kneading massage, and localized injections using various combinations of anesthetics and steroids.[58]

Thoracic Outlet Syndrome

Symptoms and signs of thoracic outlet syndrome (TOS) are not uncommon following cervical hyperextension injury. This syndrome may present with vascular and/or neurologic symptoms related to compromise of the subclavian/axillary artery/vein complex or the medial cord of the brachial plexus within the thoracic

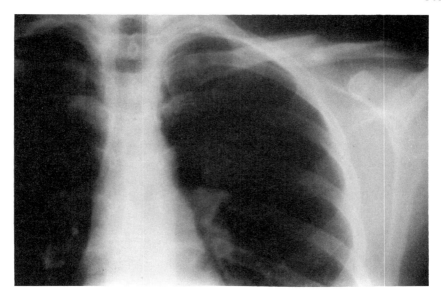

FIGURE 6. Fracture of clavical secondary to shoulder strap trauma associated with symptoms of a thoracic outlet syndrome.

outlet (Fig. 6). Although its etiology is multifactorial when associated with accidents, structural abnormalities rarely can be identified by x-rays or electrodiagnostic testing. Symptoms are aggravated by passive arm abduction with a notable concurrent decrease in radial pulse associated with the onset of bruit over the subclavian artery.[33] Typical complaints include neck, shoulder, and arm pain, inferomedial scapular pain, and tenderness in the axilla to digital palpation as well as tenderness over the ulnar nerve at the elbow. "Weakness," cramping, and/or tiredness of the arm in abduction and "numbness" of the ring and little fingers can also be experienced. An EMG demonstrating medial cord neuropathy as either slowing of ulnar nerve conduction velocity across the outlet with C8-T1 root stimulus and/or a delayed upper extremity SEP can be diagnostic. However, if these tests are normal, they do not preclude the presence of a TOS that is primarily vascular.[61] The symptoms of a TOS may be difficult to distinguish from those of a myofascial syndrome or other soft tissue injuries (Fig. 7). In both instances cervical traction often increases pain. Although a regimen of exercise has been recommended in TOS, over time rest and the avoidance of activity in a position of shoulder abduction may prove to be more productive. Infrequently, surgical resection of the first rib can be recommended.[59]

Shoulder and Arm Pain

Referred radicular pain to the shoulder, particularly the discomfort of a post-traumatic C6 root syndrome, can functionally affect the normal mechanics at the shoulder joint. Compensatory alterations in glenohumoral joint dynamics may predispose the stabilizing structure of this joint to undue stress. Most vulnerable in this regard are the rotator cuff and the associated subdeltoid bursa, the long head of the biceps tendon, and the acromioclavicular joint.

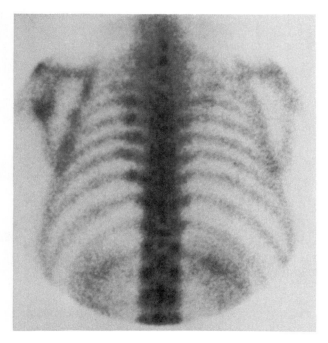

FIGURE 7. Delayed radionuclide tracer accumulation in the left 4th through 9th posterior ribs suggesting resolving fractures with normal antecedent x-ray examination.

An acute subdeltoid bursitis can be recognized by an exacerbation of pain in the subacromial area by internal and external rotation of the glenohumeral joint at 110° of shoulder abduction, with the discomfort often referred to the deltoid insertion. A bicepital tendonitis can be digitally palpated, with pain increased by resisted forearm supination. Acromioclavicular pain is often associated with crepitus, which can be both heard and palpated throughout the shoulder girdle.[6] Infrequently, a dislocation of the proximal and/or distal clavicular joint can occur secondary to local seat-belt trauma.

In the older patient a lack of shoulder joint motion can rapidly and often subtly induce the development of shoulder periarthrosis. In this regard, treatment should be aggressive, with the use of appropriate anesthetic/steroid injections, nonsteroidal anti-inflammatory agents, analgesics, ultrasound followed by hydroculator packing, assisted range of motion with stretching, and a daily active shoulder mobility program. Intermittent cervical traction is also appropriate when the symptoms of radiculopathy are also present.[60]

In addition to the thoracic outlet syndrome, another common traumatic neuropathy of the upper extremity includes the **carpal tunnel syndrome.** In both instances proximal shoulder and neck pain radiation can occur.[41] Conversely, the presence of of a post-traumatic cervical radiculopathy can mask the presence of a carpal tunnel syndrome following acute hyperextension of the wrist and hand on the steering wheel. The localized trauma can precipitate both a flexor tendon synovitis and/or median nerve neuropathy at the wrist.[22] Once clinically suspected, the presence of a carpal tunnel can be confirmed by electroneuromyography.

Initial treatment includes wrist splinting and, when appropriate, steroid injections. When conservative treatment fails, surgical section of the carpal ligament should be considered.[28] If a concomitant wrist fracture is suspected and cannot be confirmed by x-ray, a bone scan should be obtained.

Lumbar Pain

When the impacted vehicle is struck from behind, hyperextension of the torso on the pelvis also occurs as the car seat is thrust forward. In the circumstance where the driver is caught unaware, lumbar-pain complaints, particularly those associated with the sacroiliac joints, can be as disabling as intractable neck pain. In those special instances when the driver is forewarned of an impending rear impact, associated radicular right leg pain may occur. The lumbar roots already tethered in the breaking leg by knee extension may be further stretched as the torso is propelled forward on a seat-belt–restrained pelvis.[35]

Alone, acute sacroiliitis can be managed effectively by the judicious use of nonsteroidal anti-inflammatory agents, diathermy, therapeutic exercises, and when necessary steroid-Xylocaine injections. When accompanied by radicular complaints, a trial of split-table intermittent pelvic traction following thermotherapy may also be appropriate.[34]

SUMMARY

The term "whiplash" has gained widespread acceptance among the laity and the legal community both for its euphonic as well as descriptive qualities. However, as a medical synonym it continues to languish in favor of the more accepted but also more cumbersome acceleration-hyperextension cervical spine injury. In either instance the pain and subsequent disability remain the same. Expeditious and appropriate treatment continue to depend on an accurate anatomical-pathologic diagnosis and an appropriate therapeutic regimen.

REFERENCES

1. Accident Facts–1980 Edition. Chicago, National Safety Council, 1980, pp 6, 13, 42, 44, 59, 62.
2. Behrman S: Migraine as sequela of blunt head injury. Injury 9:74–76, 1977.
3. Behrman S: Traumatic neuropathy of second cervical spinal nerves. Br Med J (Clin Res) 1983:1313–1313, 1983.
4. Borrks SH, Nahum AM, Siegel AW: Causes of injury in motor vehicle accidents. Surg Gynecol Obstet 131:185–197, 1970.
5. Cailliet R: Soft Tissue Pain and Disability, 2nd ed. Philadelphia, FA Davis, 1988, pp 123–169.
6. Cailliet R: Soft Tissue Pain and Disability, 2nd ed. Philadelphia, FA Davis, 1988, pp 179–208.
7. Cain CM, Ryan GA, Fraser R, Potter G: Cervical spine injuries in road traffic crashes in South Australia. Aust NZ J Surg 59:15–19, 1989.
8. Clemens HJ, Burrow K: Experimental investigation on injury mechanism of cervical spine at frontal and rear frontal vehicle impacts. In 16th Stapp Car Crash Conference Proceedings. New York, Society of Automotive Engineers, 1972, pp 96–104.
9. Conlin PD: Whiplash revisited. Contemp Orthop 6:79–84, 1983.
10. Colachis SC Jr, Strohm BR: Effect of duration of intermittent cervical traction on vertebral separation. Arch Phys Med Rehabil 47:353–359, 1966.
11. Council on Scientific Affairs: Automobile—related injuries. JAMA 249:3216–3222, 1983.
12. Crosby EC: Corrrelative Anatomy of the Nervous System. New York, Macmillan, 1962, pp 79–80.
13. Dawes RF, Smallwood JA, Taylor I: Seatbelt injury to the female breast. Br J Surg 73:106–107, 1986.
14. Deans GT, Magalliard JN, Kerr M, Rutherford WH: Neck sprain—a major cause of disability following car accidents. Injury 18:10–12, 1987.
15. Ehne G: Extradural spinal cord and nerve root compression from benign lesions of the cervical area. In Youmans JR (ed): Neurological Surgery. Philadelphia, WB Saunders, 1982, pp 2574–2612.

16. Evans PD, Mackie IG: Fracture of the body of the sternum associated with the use of static seatbelts. Injury 16:4485–486, 1986.

17. Fakhoury GW, Gibson JR: Seatbelt hazards in pregnancy. Br J Obstet Gynaecol 93:395–396, 1986.

18. Fuentes JM, Bloncourt J, Bourbotte G: Chance's fracture. Neurochirurgie 30:113–118, 1984.

19. Greene JC, Louie R, Wycoff SJ: Preventive dentistry. JAMA 263:421–425.

20. Graham DI, Adams JH, Gennarelli TA: Pathology of brain damage in head injury. In Cooper PR (ed): Head Injury, 2nd ed. Baltimore, Williams & Wilkins, 1987, pp 72–88.

21. Gotten N: Survey of one hundred cases of whiplash injury after settlement of litigation. JAMA 162:865–867, 1956.

22. Guyon MA, Honet JC: Carpal tunnel syndrome or trigger finger associated with neck injury in automobile accidents. Arch Phy Med Rehabil 58:325–367, 1977.

23. Hamilton JR, Dearden C, Rutherford WHH Myocardial contusion associated with fracture of the sternum—Important features of the seatbelt syndrome. Injury 16:155–156, 1984.

24. Hinoki M, Niki H: Neurotological studies on the role of the sympathetic nervous system in the formation of traumatic vertigo of cervical origin. Acta Otolaryngol 330(Suppl):185–196, 1975.

25. Halliwell M, Robertson JC, Todd GB, Lobb M: Bilateral vocal cord paralysis due to whiplash injury. Br Med J (Clin Res) 288:1876–1877, 1984.

26. Heulke DF, Nusholtz GS: Cervical spine biomechanics: A review of the literature. J Orthop Res 4:232–245, 1986.

27. Hunter CR, Mayfield FH: Role of the upper cervical root in the production of pain in the head. Am J Surg 78:743–749, 1949.

28. Johnson EW: Carpal tunnel syndrome. In Johnson EW: Practical Electromyography, 2nd ed. Baltimore, Williams & Wilkins, 1988, pp 187–205.

29. Juhl M, Seerup KK: Cervical spine injuries—epidemiological investigation, medical and social consequences. Proceedings of the 6th International Conference on Biomechanics of Impacts, Bron, France, IRCOBI, 1981.

30. Kallieris D, Mattern R, Schmidt G, Warth D: Kinematic and spinal columnar injuries in active and passive passenger protection: Results of simulated frontal collisions. In Proceedings of the 1984 International Conference on Biomechanics of Impact. Bron, France, IRCOBI, 1984, pp 279–295.

31. Karbi OA, Caspari DA, Tator CH: Extrication, immobilization and radiologic investigation of patients with cervical spine injuries. Can Med Assoc J 139:817–821, 1988.

32. Kraft GH, Johnson EW, LaBan MM: The fibrositis syndrome. Arch Phys Med Rehabil 49:155–162, 1968.

33. Kurz LT: The differential diagnosis of cervical radiculopathy. In Herkowitz HN: Seminars in Spinal Surgery. Philadelphia, WB Saunders, 1989, pp 194–199.

34. LaBan MM: The lumbosacral pain syndrome. In Kaplan PE (ed): The Practice of Physical Medicine. Springfield, Charles C. Thomas, 1984, pp 107–160.

35. LaBan MM: Lumbosacral spine. In Tintinalli JE, Krome RL, Ruiz E (eds): Emergency Medicine: A Comprehensive Study Guide, 2nd ed. New York, McGraw-Hill, 1988, pp 644–649.

36. LaBan MM: Electrodiagnosis in cervical radicular and myelopathic syndromes. In Herkowitz HN: Seminars in Spinal Surgery. Philadelphia, WB Saunders, 1989, pp 222–228.

37. LaBan MM: Neck pain. In Tintinalli JE, Krome RL, Ruiz E (eds): Emergency Medicine: A Comprehensive Study Guide, 2nd ed. New York, McGraw-Hill, 1988, pp 644–649.

38. LaBan MM, Meerschaert JR: Quadriplegia following cervical traction in patients with occult epidural prosthetic metastasis. Arch Phys Med Rehabil 56:455–458, 1975.

39. LaBan M, Meerschaert JR, Johnstone KS: Carotid bruits: Their significance in the cervical radicular syndrome. Arch Phys Med Rehabil 59:34–36, 1978.

40. LaBan MM, Meerschaert JR, Taylor RS: Breast pain: A symptom of cervical radiculopathy. Arch Phys Med Rehabill 60:315–317, 1979.

41. LaBan MM, Zemenick GA, Meerschaert JR: Neck and shoulder pain: Presenting symptoms of carpal tunnel syndrome. Mich Med J 74:549–550, 1975.

42. Larder DR, Twiss MK, Mackay GM: Neck injury to car occupants using seat belts. 29th Annual Proceedings of Am Assoc Auto Med, 1985.

43. Lieberman JS: Cervical soft tissue injuries and cervical disc disease. In Leek JC, Gershwin ME, Fowler WM (eds): Principles of Physical Medicine and Rehabilitation in the Musculoskeletal Diseases. Orlando, Grune & Strattion, 1986, pp 263–286.

44. Macnab I: Acceleration injuries of the cervical spine. J Bone Joint Surg 46A:1797–1799, 1964.

45. Macnab I: The "whiplash syndrome." Orthop Clin North Am 2:389–4403, 1971.

46. Mills H, Horne G: Whiplash—manmade disease? NZ Med J 99:373–374, 1986.
47. Norris SH, Watt I: The prognosis of neck injuries resulting from rear-end vehicle collisions. J Bone Joint Surg 65B:608–611, 1983.
48. Olney DB, Marsden AK: The effect of head restraints and seat belts on the incidence of neck injury in car accidents. Injury 17:365–367, 1986.
49. Pang LQ: Neurotological aspects of whiplash injuries. Laryngoscope 81:1381–1387, 1971.
50. Polen MR, Friedman GD: Automobile injury: Selected risk factors and prevention in the health care setting. JAMA 259:76–80, 1988.
51. Porter KM: Neck sprains after car accidents. Br Med J 298:973–974, 1989.
52. Roydhouse RH: Torquing of the neck and jaw due to belt restraint in whiplash-type accidents. Lancet 1:1341, 1985.
53. Schneider RC, Schemm GW: Vertebral artery insufficiency in acute and chronic spinal trauma. J Neurosurg 18:348–360, 1961.
54. Selecki BR: Whiplash. Aust Fam Phys 13:243–247, 1984.
55. Sumchai A, Eliastam M, Werner P: Seatbelt cervical injury in an intersection type vehicular collision. J Trauma 28:1384–1388, 1988.
56. Taylor AR: The mechanism of injury to the spinal cord in the neck without damage to the vertebral column. J Bone Joint Surg 33B:543–547, 1951.
57. Toglia JU: Acute flexion-extension injury of the neck. Neurology 26:808–814, 1976.
58. Travell JG, Simons DG: Myofascial pain and dysfunction. In The Trigger Point Manual. Baltimore, Williams & Wilkins, 1983.
59. Urschel HC, Razzuk MA: Management of the thoracic-outlet syndrome: Current concepts. N Engl J Med 286:1140–1144, 1972.
60. Weiss JJ: Intraarticular steroids in the treatment of rotator cuff tear: Reappraisal by arthrography. Arch Phys Med REhabil 62:555–557, 1981.
61. Wilbourne AJ: Slowing across the thoracic outlet with thoracic outlet syndrome: Fact or fiction. Neurology 34:143, 1983.
62. Wolf RA: Four facets of automotive crash injury research. NY State J Med 66:1798–1813, 1966.

JOSEPH P. FARRELL, MS, PT

CERVICAL PASSIVE MOBILIZATION TECHNIQUES:

The Australian Approach

From Redwood Orthopaedic
Physical Therapy, Inc.
Castro Valley, California;
Senior Clinical Faculty
Kaiser Orthopedic Physical
Therapy Residency Program,
Hayward, California

Special thanks to
Carol Jo Tichenor, PT for her
considerable help in editing
this article.

Reprint requests to:
Joseph P. Farrell, MS, PT
Redwood Orthopaedic Physical
Therapy, Inc.
20211 Patio Dr., Suite 205
Castro Valley, CA 94546

Passive movement techniques are an important aspect of the total physical therapy program for patients with symptoms of cervical origin. Passive movement techniques include massage of the soft tissues, manually sustained or rhythmically applied muscle stretching, traction applied in the longitudinal axis of the cervical spine, specific or general high-velocity manipulation, and passive joint mobilization. Grieve[22] defines joint mobilization as passive, repetitive, oscillatory movements that are controllable by the patient. Joint mobilization techniques are applied to regions of the cervical spine or to specific vertebral motion segments by the hands, fingers, or thumbs of the physical therapist. The goal of passive joint mobilization is to restore full painless joint mobility to the involved vertebral motion segment.

The detailed process of evaluation that precedes the application of passive joint mobilization is unique to manual therapy, which is a subspecialty of physical therapy. Recent research[24] has pointed out that trained manual therapists are as accurate as controlled diagnostic blocks in identifying cervical zygoapophyseal joint dysfunction. The skillful hands and decision-making skills of highly trained manual therapists can assist the physician in confirming the medical diagnosis and, subsequently, in directing the patient through the process of rehabilitation. This chapter focuses on the evaluation process that leads to the successful application of cervical passive mobilization techniques as a component of the rehabilitation of the patient experiencing neck and/or arm pain of cervical origin. A brief review of schools of thought and clinical rationale of cervical mobilization techniques is presented. This forms the basis for a discussion of the examination process and selection of techniques for treatment.

Many concepts presented in this chapter are based upon the Australian approach, since the author's background in the manual therapies was influenced by the philosophies of Geoffrey Maitland. Maitland[36] was a pioneer in the development of a methodical examination for the selection of passive movement techniques.

SCHOOLS OF THOUGHT

The application of cervical mobilization procedures within the field of physical therapy is diverse. Cyriax[8] utilizes a sequence of techniques that are high-velocity procedures performed under strong traction. His early work in manual medicine formed the basis of the physical examination that is common to many philosophies within the field of manual therapy.

Kaltenborn[25] employs techniques based upon kinematic principles. His screening examination forms the basis for treatment planning. Distraction of the vertebral motion segment is often used as a trial treatment. Kaltenborn has also integrated other osteopathic, proprioceptive neuromuscular facilitatory (PNF) techniques and modalities into the treatment program to restore, as needed, normal movement to the motion segment. The McKenzie[37] approach is based upon the concepts of mechanical origin of spinal pain and patient self-treatment. Stevens and McKenzie[47] have outlined McKenzie's classification of spinal pain into three syndromes of posture, dysfunction, and derangement. The key to this approach is the manual therapist assisting the patient in learning which movements and postures produce pain and which eliminate their pain. Through patient education, exercise, and prophylaxis, the patient learns to manage his or her particular problem. The manual therapist utilizes passive movement techniques only on patients who are unable to manage their cervical complaint with self-treatment techniques. McKenzie believes that if patients are instructed to manage their own pain, then long-term benefit may be obtained.

Maitland[36] emphasizes the importance of detail in examination. The precise area and the relationship of associated symptoms form the basis for the use of standard test procedures. Movements that provoke and/or eliminate the patient's complaint are discovered by testing physiological, combined movements and adverse mechanical neural tension, and by detailed palpation of the cervical spine. The analysis of different kinds of pain and stiffness assists the manual therapist in selection of passive movement techniques. If the manual therapist is able to reproduce the patient's complaint, then the complaint may be eliminated by the passive movement technique that reproduces the patient's complaint.

Continuous assessment and skillful communication skills are key in successfully treating and progressing patients. This approach offers tremendous flexibility in choosing appropriate treatment techniques that "fit" the patient's clinical picture, not the clinicians philosophical bias.

In addition to passive joint mobilization techniques, patient education, exercise, muscle stretching, modalities, and traction are integrated into the system. The flexibility and continuous assessment process also makes possible the integration of numerous osteopathic techniques, including muscle energy[39] and counterstrain,[23] various forms of exercise, and the techniques discovered by McKenzie and Kaltenborn.

CLINICAL RATIONALE OF CERVICAL MOBILIZATION TECHNIQUES

Most patients who seek treatment for symptoms of cervical origin are usually functionally limited by pain. The goal of treatment then revolves around eliminating or minimizing symptoms so that the patient is able to return to a functionally normal lifestyle. Patients suitable for treatment by passive movement techniques are those whose symptoms are aggravated by activity and selected postures, and are relieved be rest and other antalgic postures.

Manual therapists often treat patients complaining of symptoms such as pain, numbness, tingling, burning sensations, heaviness, and coldness of the upper extremity. These symptoms are commonly related to cervical spondylosis and subsequent nerve root disorders. Similarly, disc bulges or osteophytes of the uncovertebral region and the zygoapophyseal joints are common causative factors rather than acute disc prolapse.[40,45,50]

Considerable debate exists concerning the biomechanical rationale for passive movement treatment of painful spinal conditions. Paris[41] supports the theory that repetitive passive joint oscillations carried out at the limit of the joint's available range can have a mechanical effect upon joint mobility. These passive movements need to stretch tissues by moving into an area of plastic deformation of the stress-strain curve, or to the point of failure. This theory is consistent with the notion that periarticular structures are the major cause of restriction of joint movement.[52] Passive movement techniques performed in the correct direction at varying velocities may "snap" periarticular adhesions responsible for joint restriction.[36,38]

Mechanically controlled passive or active movements of joints have been shown to improve the rate of tendon repair and gliding function within tendon sheaths during the repair process.[51] A more intensive inflammatory reaction (healing with scar formation and muscle regeneration) has been found in mobilized compared with immobilized rats. In addition, a more parallel orientation of regenerating muscle fibers was discovered in the mobilized rats.[30]

Neurological effects of passive movement techniques include restoration of axonal transport due to mechanically induced deformation of spinal nerves,[29] stimulation of large-fiber joint afferents conveyed by joint receptors that depends on the gate control theory,[53] and stimulation of clinically effective levels of endorphins.[49]

Experienced manual therapists often report that low back pain or lower extremity pain has been provoked by palpation of the cervical or thoracic spine. This implies some neurological mediation as a hypothesis for the use of passive movement techniques. The neurological basis for passive movement treatment warrants further research to confirm the theories mentioned.

Increased levels of intra-articular pressure from high levels of intra-articular fluid or from increased muscle tension on the joint capsule[31] are possible causative factors responsible for pain and limitation of joint movement in injured or arthritic joints.[15] The cause of pain in osteoarthritic joints has been attributed to increased intraosseous pressure.[4] Arnoldi et al.[1] suggest that intraosseous pressure may be influenced by joint position and intra-articular pressure. In a small survey, Giovanelli-Blacker et al.[18] demonstrated that intra-articular pressure in lumbar zygoapophyseal joints was reduced by passive oscillations conducted at the end range of joint movement. The findings of this study suggest that end-range passive mobilization techniques may have a positive effect upon decreasing intra-articular pressures in patients exhibiting signs and symptoms related to the "degenerative cascade" affecting spinal motion segments. Furthermore, Frank et al.[16] reported that passive movement of joints stretches and lubricates tissues and induces metabolic changes in soft tissue, cartilage, and bone. This supports the use of passive movement techniques in patients who exhibit degenerative joint changes.

Manual therapists are routinely confronted with the diagnostic difficulties of differentiating the cause of shoulder and arm pain that is referred from a multitude of structures in the cervical spine. Experimental studies on humans have produced pain in the shoulder region and upper extremity by stimulation of interspinous ligaments,[14,27] cervical intervertebral discs,[6] paraspinal and scapular musculature,[26] and the cervical roots via mechanical distortion.[17] Pathological and degenerative changes that occur in the cervical spine may be accompanied by fibrosis and adhesion formation in and around nerve roots. Nerve roots are susceptible to irritation from tensile stresses arising from mechanical interfaces, such as disc bulges and osteophytes of the uncovertebral and zygoapophyseal joints, which may inhibit mobility or extensibility.

Elvey[11] developed a method of testing the mobility of cervical nerve roots and peripheral nerve extensions with a procedure called the **upper limb tension test.** This procedure combines shoulder depression, shoulder abduction, extension, lateral rotation, forearm supination and elbow extension, and wrist/finger extension. The major cervical nerve roots affected are C5, 6, whereas the median nerve peripherally is most stretched. Many clinicians in Australia have studied Elvey's maneuver and have offered modifications to the test,[5] and they have conducted studies documenting normative responses.[28] Passive mobilization techniques and their effect upon the immobility of cervical nerve roots are beyond the scope of this chapter. However, this is an important aspect of the total treatment arsenal of manual therapists. For further information, please refer to the extensive literature pertaining to the treatment of adverse mechanical neural tension signs.[3,5]

The efficacy of cervical mobilization techniques in treating cervical signs and symptoms has not been substantiated due to the paucity of controlled studies pertaining to mobilization of the cervical spine.[42,46] Considerable clinical research is, however, available pertaining to mobilization and manipulation of the lumbar spine. These studies tend to evaluate one specific treatment technique rather than study a system or philosophy of treatment. Researching a system of treatment[13] is more clinically relevant, since it is rare that the application of one technique will remedy the patient's total problem. Patients who are in acute back pain of short duration tended to respond at a faster rate when treated with passive mobilization techniques administered by a manual therapist compared with other forms of treatment.[13] Further controlled clinical research utilizing cervical passive mobilization techniques is needed to document the efficacy of passive movement techniques as a component of the rehabilitation process.

THE EXAMINATION PROCESS

The Subjective Examination

Considerable literature exists on procedures for interviewing the patient.[21,36] Key ingredients to the interview process are a personal commitment to the patient and the utilization of verbal and nonverbal communication skills. By simple questioning, active listening, clarification, and identification of what the patient feels is important, the skillful clinician should be able to determine the patient's major complaint(s) during the initial visit.

The goals of the subjective examination are presented so the reader acquires an appreciation of the detailed interview process that is required to assist the clinician in understanding the patient's major complaint. If the major complaint is not fully understood, the clinician risks applying cervical mobilization techniques inappropriately or to the wrong body region, which may endanger the patient.

The goals of the subjective component of the examination are to:

1. Obtain a patient profile that provides an understanding of the patient's lifestyle and specifics of his or her working environment.
2. Identify the major problem, such as pain, stiffness, weakness, tingling, or any functional loss.
3. Acquire a detailed description of all of the patient's symptoms and thus make an assessment of which body area(s) will receive the major emphasis during the interview and subsequent physical examination.
4. Gather sufficient information to understand how the problem affects the patient's lifestyle throughout the 24-hour day.
5. Begin to formulate a clinical working hypothesis related to the presenting disorder and progression of the disorder.
6. Determine if there are any dangers or contraindications to treatment or the use of specific techniques.
7. Assess the patient's perception of his or her problem.

The components (area of symptoms, expression of symptoms, special questions, and the history) of the subjective examination have been outlined in detail by numerous authorities.[21,36] Of importance for determining the safe use of mobilization techniques are the special question and history components. Special questions pertaining to the patient's past medical history, use of steroids, and complaints of dizziness assist the clinician in identifying contraindications to mobilization. These contraindications include malignancy involving the spinal column, signs and symptoms of spinal cord compression, active inflammatory and infective arthritic conditions, advanced stages of rheumatoid arthritis affecting the ligaments of the cervical spine, and bone diseases.[21]

Several situations necessitate caution in the application of passive mobilization techniques. In the presence of neurological signs, techniques that compromise the intervertebral foramen on the side of the painful extremity should be avoided. Osteoporosis necessitates gentle application of mobilization techniques, since loss of up to 40% of bone salts occurs prior to observable radiological evidence.[32] Previous metastatic disease in tissues other than the spine does not necessarily contraindicate passive movement treatment. Similarly, passive mobilization of the cervical spine may be performed if particular attention is paid to the history and behavior of the symptoms. Additional diagnostic testing to rule out spinal metastases is necessary if the cause of the patient's complaint is not related to movement or selected postures.

Dizziness is a common symptom associated with vertebrobasilar arterial disease (VAD). Regardless of the origin, every patient who presents with upper-quarter dysfunction should be questioned in detail concerning the presence of dizziness prior to cervical examination and treatment. Although the incidence of injury from manipulation of the cervical spine is small,[20,44] the potential danger for injury that may lead to permanent neurological damage or death cannot be overlooked when examining the patient. The incidence of injury from passive cervical mobilization techniques has not been adequately explored in the literature.

Coman[7] has outlined the major symptoms (diplopia, drop attacks, dysarthria, and dysphagia) associated with VAD, which may aid in differentiating VAD from cervical vertigo. If dizziness is an unaccompanied symptom, it remains difficult to differentiate it from VAD or from inner ear disorders that also may produce dizziness. Considerable attention should be paid to the movements that reproduce dizziness, especially rotation, extension, or combinations of these movements. Details of the subjective and objective examination of the patient who presents with symptoms of dizziness have recently been reported.[2,19]

The Physical Examination

Analysis of the information gathered from the subjective examination enables the clinician to plan the physical examination. The subjective examination assists the clinician in identifying the following:

1. Structure(s) that could be responsible for the presenting symptoms.
2. The need to examine other structures or functional movements that may assist in proving/disproving a working clinical hypothesis.
3. The irritability, nature, and stage of the disorder, which will dictate the vigor of the examination (e.g., whether to reproduce local or referred symptoms) and subsequent application of mobilization techniques.
4. Any factors that might contraindicate any portion of the physical examination.
5. Possible rationale for symptoms (e.g., lifestyle, repetitive nature of the patient's work, any other predisposing factor) so that the examination and treatment lead to total patient management, not just symptomatic relief.

The goals of the physical examination are to:

1. Identify movement patterns and restriction of movement that relate to pain-provoking and pain-easing factors reported by the patient.
2. Reproduce the patient's complaint via movement testing and palpation of the cervical or associated regions.
3. Confirm the irritability of the condition.
4. Confirm the cause of the patient's complaint based upon the subjective examination.
5. Determine the neurological status.

The focus of the physical examination will vary according to the assessment of subjective data synthesized during the plan of the physical examination. For example, if the major complaint is right, low cervical aching radiating to the radial aspect of the right wrist, then the clinician must examine the cervical spine, shoulder complex, elbow complex, wrist region, and must perform a neurological exam to determine the cause of the problem. Further tests of adverse mechanical neural tension are in order[5,11] because of the pain pattern presented.

Routine Movement Tests

Through skillful observation of the patient undressing, opening a door, or the posture with which the patient holds the head or upper extremity, much information can be learned about the severity of the disorder and the way the patient reacts to the complaint. This information is utilized to confirm the vigor of movement testing.

Traditional active anatomical plane movements (cervical flexion, extension, lateral flexion, and rotation) should be examined. The following information is important for the clinician to acquire so that reproducible baseline data are available to reassess change in movement and pain patterns as a result of a particular treatment technique[33]:

1. Resting symptoms.
2. The location and behavior of symptoms during the testing of movement.
3. The quality and duration of symptoms reproduced.
4. The effect of movement upon each related and unrelated symptom.
5. Intersegmental movement and quality of movement through range.
6. The presence of protective deformity and its relevance to the problem.
7. The effect of pressure at the end range of the normal or the pathological limit and the response to releasing pressure.

If standard active movement tests do not reproduce the patient's complaint, then the clinician should consider sustaining movements, performing repeated movements, compressing or distracting the cervical spine, performing movements under compression/distraction, altering the speed of the movement test, or performing combined movement testing.[9,10]

Combined Movement Testing

Functional movements of the spine nearly always involve a combination of anatomical plane movements. In many instances the clinician must analyze the provoking activity and break down its components to reproduce the patient's complaint. Often standard physiological movement testing does not reproduce the patient's complaint or only reproduces one component of the patient's complaint. If during the routine movement testing, a particular physiological movement reproduces the patient's complaint (primary movement), further information may be gathered to establish a movement pattern to assist in predicting the result of treatment and the manner in which both the symptoms and movement signs may improve.[9] Edwards describes regular patterns of movement that respond to treatment in a way such that the least painful movement will improve prior to the most painful movement. Figure 1 depicts a regular pattern of movement. Right lateral flexion in neutral (Fig. 1A) reproduces right low cervical pain and right lateral flexion performed in flexion (Fig. 1B) is painless. Right lateral flexion performed in extension (Fig. 1C) is most painful. Right lateral flexion in neutral will improve prior to right lateral flexion in extension. The treatment response of regular patterns tends to be more predictable. Most of the patients in the author's clinical practice present cervical complaints secondary to trauma. These tend to present with irregular movement patterns that respond to treatment in an unpredictable manner.

Examination Procedure. Explain to the patient that your goal in further movement testing is either to ease the pain if the problem is irritable or to reproduce the major complaint if the problem is nonirritable. An irritable symptom requires minimal activity to reproduce and generally takes greater than 30 minutes to settle. A nonirritable symptom generally requires a significant amount of activity (e.g., 45 min) to provoke the pain and a short period of time to settle. From the standard movement testing in neutral, the primary complaint is determined. If pain is the dominant complaint, the goal is to find the combination of movements that eases the complaint. If the primary movement is right rotation, then the patient is instructed to rotate to the right until the complaint is reproduced. The clinician then maintains right rotation and adds other physiological movements such as neck flexion (Fig. 2) in sequence while methodically assessing the pain response. Right rotation may be tested in flexion

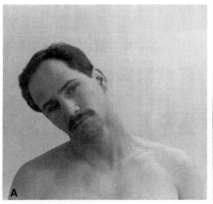
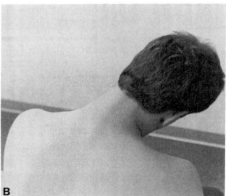
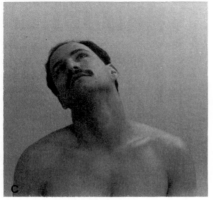

FIGURE 1. *A,* Right lateral flexion in neutral. *B,* Right lateral flexion in flexion. *C,* Right lateral flexion in extension.

and extension to assist the clinician in determining the nature of the movement pattern and, subsequently, to assist in selection of the appropriate technique.

If standard movement testing in neutral does not provoke comparable symptoms, then the clinician must analyze the activity that reproduces the complaint

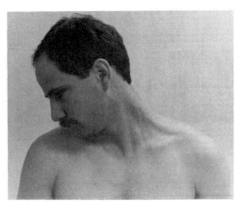

FIGURE 2. Neck flexion in right rotation.

and perform combined movements in various positions (sitting, supine, or sidelying) or couple the combined movement testing with passive accessory movement testing anteriorly or posteriorly, perform upper limb tension testing, or look to associated areas that may contribute to the total patient picture. Clinically, if right low cervical pain is aggravated by serving a tennis ball approximately 30 times, then the combined movements (Fig. 3) of cervical extension, right rotation, and right lateral flexion should be examined and the sequence of the testing changed (e.g., right lateral flexion, right rotation, and extension examined in differing orders). The symptoms may differ depending upon the sequence of testing. In addition, the shoulder complex may need to be examined. Adverse mechanical neural tension testing such as upper limb tension tests (Fig. 4)[5,11] or slump sit tests (Fig. 5)[34] may need to be performed to determine which structures are involved. Palpation of the cervical spine is of major importance, since symptoms are often not reproduced until detailed palpation is performed.

Posterior Palpation of the Cervical Spine

Palpation of the posterior aspect of the cervical spine may be the most informative aspect of the physical examination of the cervical spine.[35] Considerable information is gathered from palpation of the soft tissues, assessment of vertebral position, and movement of the vertebra via passive accessory intervertebral movement testing performed using the therapist's thumbs.

A recent study by Jull et al.[24] in Australia evaluated one manual therapist's ability to identify cervical zygoapophyseal joint syndromes in 20 patients, all of whom had complained of chronic neck pain or headaches for at least a year. Two

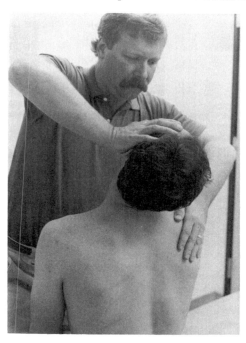

FIGURE 3. Combined movement: extension, right rotation, right lateral flexion.

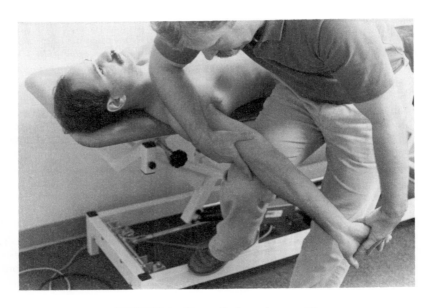

FIGURE 4.   Upper limb tension test #1.

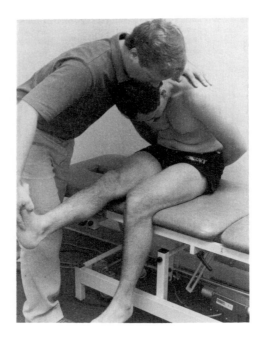

FIGURE 5.   Slump test.

research questions were proposed: (1) Can manual therapists actually sense abnormalities in the joint by palpating movements between specific vertebra? (2) Are the allegedly palpable abnormalities diagnostic or are they nonspecific signs?

The study employed a cross-over design. In one group of 11 patients, the presence or absence of a symptomatic joint was established by radiologically controlled diagnostic nerve blocks; then the patients were examined by the manual therapist 1 to 4 weeks after the nerve blocks. The manual therapist was unaware of the medical diagnosis. In the second group of 9 patients, the order of events was reversed. The manual therapist first examined the patients, gave an opinion as to whether there were symptoms present, and, if present, at what vertebral motion segment. Neither the manual therapist nor the medical team had any knowledge of the cause of the patient's symptoms.

Of the 20 patients in both groups, the manual therapist correctly identified all 15 with proven symptomatic zygoapophyseal joints and correctly specified the location of each joint. The manual therapist also correctly concluded that the other 5 patients were free of symptoms. The authors of this study[24] concluded that for the diagnosis of symptomatic cervical zygoapophyseal joints, the manual examination by a trained manual therapist is as accurate as expensive radiologically controlled diagnostic blocks. In addition, the manual therapist could not possibly have made accurate clinical diagnoses so consistently had she not in fact been able to palpate and assess the specific vertebral motion segments.

The palpation techniques utilized in the Jull study have been described in detail by Maitland[36] and are also performed as treatment techniques. These accessory movements are performed routinely along the entire spine using pressure of the thumbs. They include the following:

1. Posterior-anterior (PA) pressures on the spinous processes of the vertebral motion segment.
2. Unilateral PA pressures applied along the laminae and adjacent to the spinous processes moving laterally to the zygoapophyseal joints.
3. Transverse pressures performed against the lateral aspect of the spinous process.

The variations of these movements are endless. The position of the palpating thumbs or the direction of the movement (medial, lateral cephalad, caudad) may be altered so that the pressures placed upon the zygoapophyseal joint and the intervertebral discs are different. The palpation assessment by manual therapists with the thumbs to reproduce the most comparable symptom(s) and signs is unique to the Maitland system. It is essential in determining the correct treatment technique and in determining the directions and vigor of the technique.

Anterior Palpation of the Cervical Spine

Palpation of the anterior aspect of the cervical spine is particularly valuable in patients with the following:

1. Whiplash.
2. Anterior shoulder or arm pain, especially in the presence of a positive upper limb tension sign.
3. Shoulder pain but negative signs.
4. Hard-to-reproduce shoulder pain/arm pain.
5. Repetitive strain injury.[12]
6. Obesity, pregnancy, and/or advanced age with inability to lie prone.

Careful assessment is necessary when palpating the neck anteriorly due to the intimate relationships of the vagus nerve, subclavian artery, carotid artery, phrenic nerve, stellate ganglion, and the brachial plexus. Anterior palpation is generally not indicated in the presence of bilateral arm pain, acute irritable disc, nerve root irritations that present with muscle guarding, or in the presence of cervical fracture.

The use and application of anterior cervical mobilization techniques will be outlined in the technique section.

SELECTION OF TECHNIQUE

Maitland[36] outlines in detail specific guidelines in choosing an appropriate passive mobilization technique. Of importance are the following points:

Area of Pain/Symptoms. Symmetrical pain presentations respond to techniques that affect the motion segment in a symmetrical manner, e.g., central PA pressures, traction. Unilateral symptoms respond to techniques affecting the vertebral motion segments in an asymmetrical manner, e.g., rotation, lateral flexion, posterior unilateral PA pressures, anterior unilateral AP pressures, or combined movements.

History of Complaint. Caution is indicated with progressive conditions suggesting neurological compromise. A technique that opens the intervertebral foramen or a combined movement that does not yield compression on the side of the painful complaint is indicated, e.g., lateral flexion, rotation, traction, or pain-easing combined movement.

Selection of Most or Least Painful Technique. It is always safest to choose the position, direction, and amplitude of movement that is painless or least painful first. As the patient improves and the condition is not easily aggravated, the treatment may be progressed within the painful range if methodical assessment is practiced by the clinician.

The Disorder Often Dictates the Choice of Technique. For example, initially an acute cervical nerve root irritation is best treated with gentle static traction or the pain-easing combined movement. A chronic nerve root irritation requires treatment of joint signs (posterior or anterior unilateral pressures, rotation, combined movements, and upper limb tension stretching) to improve mobility as well as the pain pattern.

Grade of Technique. In the presence of muscle spasm, a small-amplitude mobilization short of reproduction of spasm should be utilized. Clinical experience and previously mentioned neurological effects suggest that end-range passive mobilizations performed in the combined movement position of most comfort are beneficial.

Speed and Rhythm of Technique. Where pain dominates or spasm is a factor, slow, smooth rhythmical oscillations are most comfortable and successful. Sustained techniques are useful when symptoms are reproduced by sustained postures.

Amount of Treatment. This is dependent upon whether pain or stiffness is the predominant factor. In the painful condition, one or two 20-second applications of a technique are all the patient may be able to tolerate. In the patient whose stiffness is dominant, multiple bouts and techniques may be indicated. Greater than one treatment technique is generally used when two unrelated areas of pain require treatment or the stiffness of multiple vertebral motion segments are contributing to the patient's complaint. The manual therapist must assess all relevant movement signs and symptoms between techniques to **validate** each technique.

The rules of selection of technique evolve from the experience of each manual therapist. Creative manual therapists use their past experience to improvise instinctively in achieving the optimal end result, often at times when most clinicians give up on the patient. Some commonly used procedures will be presented so that the reader may gain an understanding of the nature and application of these passive mobilization techniques. The creative manual therapist in practice may use thousands of variations of these techniques to achieve the desired goal(s).

The following techniques have been previously described by Maitland[36] and Edwards.[9,10]

PASSIVE ACCESSORY TECHNIQUES

Central Posterior-Anterior (PA) Pressures

The pads of the thumb tips rest upon the spinous process while the hands encompass the soft tissues of the neck and head of the vertebra to be mobilized (Fig. 6). The technique is performed in a controlled manner by a rhythmical

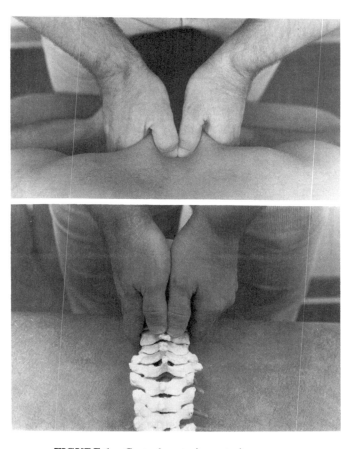

FIGURE 6. Central posterior-anterior pressure.

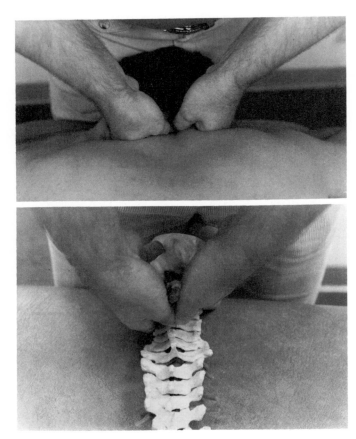

FIGURE 7.   Central posterior-anterior pressure directed cephalad.

oscillatory pressure applied to the spinous process. If the patient is experiencing considerable pain, the technique may be modified. The palmar surfaces of the fingers lift the neck into varying degrees of flexion, allowing the depth of the mobilization to be performed in the pain-free range of available movement.

Application.   The use of central PA pressure is of considerable value in those patients who present with midline or bilaterally distributed head, neck, or arm pain related to cervical spondylotic changes. **Variations** of the technique include angulating the central PA pressure cephalad (Fig. 7), caudad (Fig. 8), right or left (Fig. 9), and in combination (e.g., caudad/right-directed PA pressures [Fig. 10]), depending upon palpation findings. Clinically, if caudad/right-directed PA pressures at C5, 6 reproduce a patient's major complaint of chronic medial-border scapular pain and the patient is not responding to other forms of treatment—e.g., soft-tissue massage, central PAs at C5, 6, and stabilization training—then it would be reasonable to change the treatment to a PA caudad/right-directed technique. Initially the technique should be performed in the pain-free portion of the available range of motion for each vertebral segment. As pain-free range of motion improves, the technique is progressed further into the available

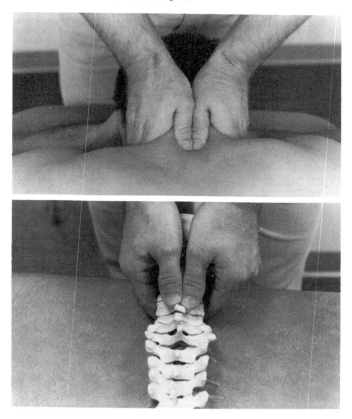

FIGURE 8.   Central posterior-anterior pressure directed caudad.

range for that particular segment, until joint mobility is restored and painless. Maitland's[36] grading system is employed to communicate the depth, amplitude, and vigor of the technique.

The patient who presents with stiffness into right rotation or right lateral flexion often has multiple vertebral motion segments contributing to the lack of mobility. Generally, passive accessory movements such as central PA pressures achieve quicker results when performed in the position of greatest stiffness (e.g., central PA pressure performed in right lateral flexion, Fig. 11). Clinically, this approach is also used in treating stiff peripheral joint disorders such as frozen-shoulder syndrome.

Unilateral Posterior-Anterior Pressures

The physical therapist stands to the side of the patient's head and places the tips of the thumbs on the posterior surface of the zygoapophyseal joint, while the hands conform to the soft tissues of the neck (Fig. 12). Care must be taken to grasp the neck gently but firmly so as to not slip off the articular process. The oscillatory unilateral PA pressure over the zygoapophyseal joint should produce a nodding action of the head if performed correctly.

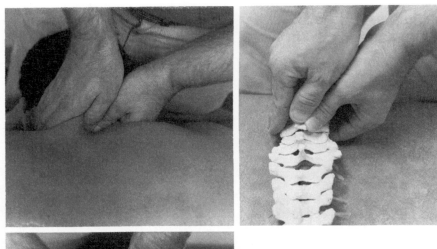

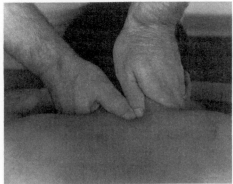

FIGURE 9. *(top left and right).* Central posterior-anterior pressure directed left.

FIGURE 10 *(bottom left).* Central posterior-anterior pressure directed right caudad.

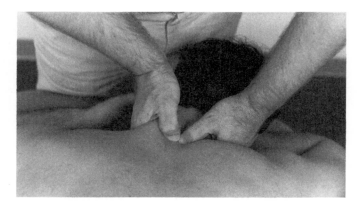

FIGURE 11.   Central posterior-anterior pressure in right lateral flexion.

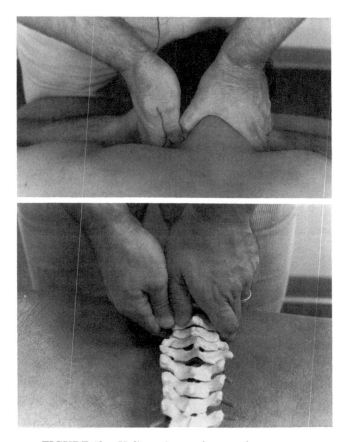

FIGURE 12.   Unilateral posterior-anterior pressure.

Application.   This technique is used in patients who present with unilateral headache, or cervical, upper thoracic, or arm complaints. **Variations** of this technique include directing the pressure medially (Fig. 13) when the joint is very stiff and pain is minimal. This variation is of particular value when treating headaches of C2, 3 origin.[36,48] Laterally directed unilateral PAs (Fig. 14) are employed when firm pressure over the zygoapophyseal joint is very painful. As described in a previous section, unilateral PAs may be combined with physiological movements to treat stiffness.

Anterior-Posterior (AP) Unilateral Pressure
With the patient supine, the physical therapist sits or stands by the patient's head with a broad-based thumb contact over the anterior tubercle of the transverse process of the vertebral motion segment to be treated (Fig. 15). Caution should be exercised to gradually sink through the anterior soft tissues of the neck, since bone on bone contact is uncomfortable. Often the muscle belly at some levels needs to be moved to one side to gain access to the desired portion of the most symptomatic vertebral motion segment. At times, palpating toward

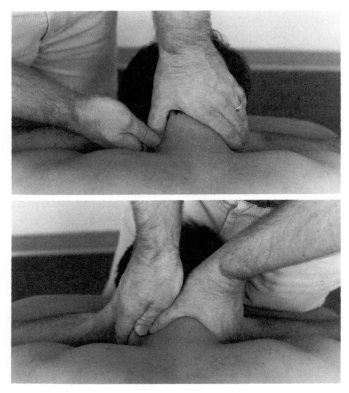

FIGURE 13 *(top).*   Unilateral posterior-anterior pressure directed medially.

FIGURE 14. *(bottom).*   Unilateral posterior-anterior pressure directed laterally.

the midline over the intervertebral disc may be required to find the vertebral motion segment that requires treatment. The technique is performed by rhythmical oscillatory movements of the thumb. The movement is produced by the physical therapist's arms.

   Application.   Use of this technique has been previously outlined in the anterior palpation section. AP unilateral pressures are frequently used in patients with arm/shoulder pain and those with positive upper limb tension signs. It is applicable from C1 to T2, 3 in most individuals.

   Variations of AP unilaterals include angulating the pressures as outlined for previous techniques. The most common variation in application of AP unilateral pressures is combining cervical physiological movements in an effort to "turn off" the pain. For example, if AP unilateral pressure at C5, 6 reproduces local low cervical neck pain that radiates to the anterior upper forearm, then the manual therapist seeks the physiological movement that enables the painless performance of AP unilateral C5, 6. Often lateral flexion or rotation toward the side of the pain allows the painless performance of the AP unilateral pressure (Fig. 16). As the patient progresses, the principles of combined movements are used, in that the treatment is performed within the patient's pain-free range of motion. Generally, less lateral flexion (Fig. 17) or rotation will be required. End range of

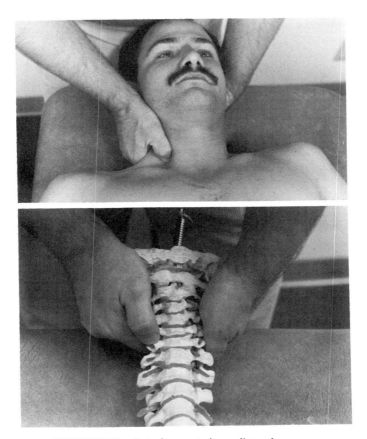

FIGURE 15. Anterior-posterior unilateral pressure.

movements is also used, since the technique is performed into stiffness but in a painless manner. Often by angulating cephlad or caudad anteriorly on a symptomatic vertebral motion segment, the angulation at the particular symptomatic segment may be painless. Again, the most painless direction and position are chosen for the initial application of the technique.

PASSIVE PHYSIOLOGICAL MOVEMENT TECHNIQUES

Cervical Rotation (Localized to the Left, C2, 3)

The patient is positioned supine with the head/neck extending beyond the end of the treatment table. If the C2, 3 zygoapophyseal joint on the right is the symptomatic vertebral motion segment, the manual therapist stands on the patient's right while cradling the head with the left arm and left upper chest region. The left hand cups the chin. The therapist's right proximal phalanx of the index finger subtly takes up the skin slack over the C2, 3 interspinous space and laterally rests over the right C3, 3 zygoapophyseal joint. The neck is then flexed/extended to find the mid-range for the C2, 3 zygoapophyseal joint. While maintaining the midrange flexion/extension at C2, 3, the therapist rotates the

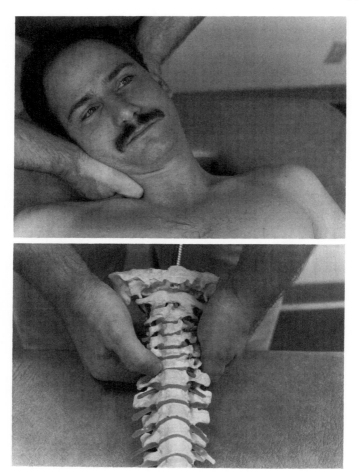

FIGURE 16.   Anterior-posterior unilateral pressure in right lateral flexion.

head to the left until the C2, 3 zygoapophyseal joint tightens under the proximal phalanx of the index finger (manual contact on occiput for generalized rotational technique). The technique is performed via gentle oscillatory rotational movements to the left, with simultaneous movement of the therapist's arms. The head moves in an oscillatory manner around the vertical axis (Fig. 18).

Application.   The technique is applied in the presence of unilateral symptoms of cervical origin and when opening of the intervertebral foramen is desired for upper extremity symptoms. It is most successful when rotating away from the side of the pain. In the presence of a positive upper limb tension test, rotation away from the side of pain often provokes pain. Therefore, rotation towards the side of pain may be indicated. **Variations** include performing the technique in sitting if the patient is unable to lie supine or if the desired changes are not obtained supine. This technique may also be performed regionally with manual contact of the therapist's right hand on the occiput rather than over the right

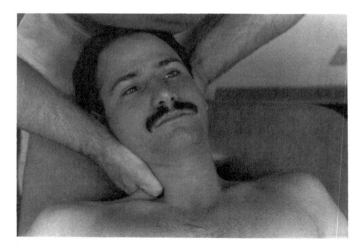

FIGURE 17.   Anterior-posterior unilateral pressure in less lateral flexion.

zygoapophyseal joint. Generalized rotations are used when the posterior aspect of the neck is too tender to touch or when multiple motion segments require mobilization due to stiffness. Special care should be exercised in the presence of dizziness, as noted previously in the subjective examination section.

Cervical Lateral Flexion (Localized to the Right)

The patient position and manual contacts by the clinician are as previously described for localized rotation. The therapist's left forearm is adjusted so it lies almost under the occiput while the right hand is moved over the right ear. The proximal phalanx of the right index rests against the zygoapophyseal joint of the vertebral motion segment to be treated. The physical therapist moves along side

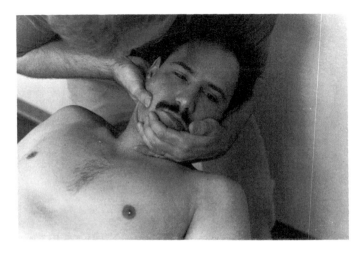

FIGURE 18.   Cervical rotation (localized to the right C2,3).

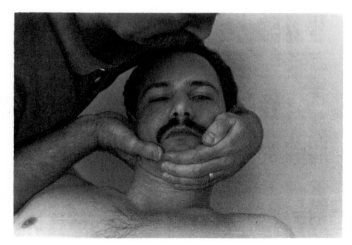

FIGURE 19.   Cervical lateral flexion (localized to the right).

the patient's right shoulder so that the physical therapist's right arm lies over the patient's right shoulder. Mid-range between flexion/extension is palpated with the right proximal phalanx. The head is laterally flexed to the right with the left hand while the right hand slightly displaces the head to the left. By firmly supporting the head and neck, an oscillatory lateral flexion movement is produced by the rocking movement of the physical therapist's hips. Simultaneously, the neck is displaced away from the therapist. The movement is a pure lateral flexion localized to the desired motion segment by firm pressure against the articular pillar (Fig. 19).

Application.   Use of this technique is similar to that of cervical rotation. It is best employed in the presence of unilateral symptoms of cervical origin that radiate into the arm, head, or scapular regions. It is most successful when laterally flexing the neck away from the side of pain. In the presence of stiffness and no distal symptoms, it is safe to laterally flex *toward* the side of pain after a trial of laterally flexing *away* from the side of pain. Often, active cervical rotation improves after lateral flexion mobilization. **Variations** of this technique are dependent upon the region of the neck to be treated. For example, more cervical flexion is required to treat the low cervical region compared to the upper cervical region. The passive mid-range between flexion/extension varies from upper to the lower cervical spine.

COMBINED MOVEMENT TECHNIQUES

Combined movement techniques are complicated to assess and apply. An example follows: Left cervical rotation is the primary movement reproducing left low cervical pain, and it is least painful when performed in flexion (sitting) compared to left rotation in flexion performed in a supine position. The initial choice of treatment position is sitting. Treatment progression is related to changing position rather than changing the grade of the movement. Therefore, in this example, the patient would be initially treated with left lateral flexion performed in flexion. As the patient improves, the left rotation would be performed more toward the neutral or extended position in a pain-free range. Two techniques are described that may be performed in supine or sitting depending on the therapist's evaluation.

Left Rotation in Flexion C5, 6 (Sitting)

The physical therapist places the pad of the right index finger on the right hand side of the spinous process of C6, while the right middle finger and thumb are placed over the articular process of C6. This allows for stabilization of C6. The little finger of the left hand rests over the C5 vertebral motion segment and over the spinous processes of the vertebra above. The spine is flexed down to the C5, 6 motion segment, then left rotation is performed in an oscillatory fashion so that C5 rotates to the left on C6 (Fig. 20). The manual therapist must make sure, via questioning, that the technique is performed in a pain-free range.

Flexion in Left Rotation C5, 6 (Sitting)

The manual contact for stabilizing C6 is the same as described for the previous technique. The left arm is held around the forehead with caution so as not to compress the head with the biceps. The left arm and the pad of the left little finger are placed over the inferior facet of C5. With the left arm, the head is rotated until maximum left rotation is palpated at C5, 6. The right index finger is placed on the superior tip of the spinous process of C6. The pad of the little finger is then hooked under the inferior aspect of the spinous process of C5. The mobilization of flexion performed in left rotation is carried out by abducting the left arm so that the head moves in a nodding fashion while maintaining stabilization of C6 (Fig. 21). If the technique is pain-producing, the rotation or flexion component may need to be altered to achieve painless performance of the technique.

HOW PASSIVE MOBILIZATION TECHNIQUES FIT INTO THE TOTAL CLINICAL PICTURE

The success of any rehabilitation program hinges upon accurate assessment of the patient's functional limitations as they relate to his/her lifestyle and work

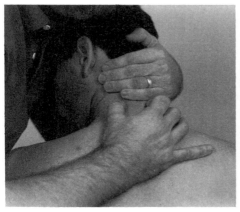 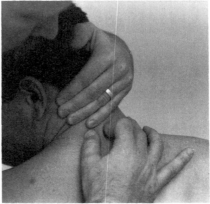

FIGURE 20 *(left).*   Left rotation in flexion C5,6 (sitting).

FIGURE 21 *(right).*   Flexion in left rotation C5,6 (sitting).

environment. From this assessment, realistic goals are set to achieve the desired treatment outcome. Of equal importance is the necessity to continuously reassess the effect of each modality, exercise, or treatment technique so that the changing nature of the patient's problem is appreciated. Continual reassessment assists the clinician in determining the validity of the treatment technique(s) of choice and yields information as to which structures are most likely contributing to the patient's complaint.

During the initial phase of rehabilitation, control of pain and the inflammatory process is necessary. The application of gentle passive mobilization techniques to the appropriate vertebral motion segment(s) may be helpful to improve segmental mobility and functional range of motion, and to decrease pain. As the patient's functional range of motion and pain pattern improves (e.g., cervical rotation), the mobilization technique will be performed further into the available range of motion for that segment. The technique is continued until movement is painless or no functional change is detected. In the presence of both joint and soft tissue limitation, the manual therapist should assess the effect of the joint mobilization technique upon the soft tissue component. If there is little or no change in the soft tissue component, then specific muscle stretching or the soft tissue massage techniques should be applied to change the soft tissue component of the condition. Likewise, if an element of adverse mechanical neural tension is present, the effects of joint mobilization and/or soft tissue muscle stretching upon the tension sign must be assessed. If no change is noted, specific techniques that treat adverse mechanical neural tension should be utilized to address it as a component of the total clinical picture. Modalities such as ice and transcutaneous electrical nerve stimulation (TENS) may be used in conjunction with various manual therapy techniques as long as the value of the modality is assessed. If anti-inflammatory medications have been prescribed by the physician as an adjunct to treatment during the inflammatory phase of treatment, they should also be assessed.

As the irritability of the cervical complaint decreases and the functional range of cervical motion improves, specific exercises to strengthen and stretch the neck, thoracic region, and upper extremity musculature often assist in maintaining cervical mobility. The mobility of cervical musculature is important, since shortened muscles lead to joint limitations that may facilitate a pain cycle that is difficult to break.[43] If the patient is suffering from chronic cervical dysfunction, the concurrent use of joint mobilization with muscle stretching and exercise is required to address all components of the multifactoral problem. Furthermore, instruction in body mechanics and self-treatment techniques is of importance so that dependence upon the physical therapist is not fostered.

Specific training of the patient is required when repetitive tasks are performed at work and during recreational activities. In this instance endurance and coordination should be addressed in the rehabilitation program and should be sport- or job-specific. Commonplace in physical therapy clinics are pulley systems, free weights, stationary bikes, gym balls, and assorted household items that are used for functional training of the patient. Equipment of this nature is easily adaptable and inexpensive for patients to use for long-term management through home exercise programs.

There are some patients who have not responded to treatment with modalities and specific stabilization exercises aimed at strengthening and stretching the neck and associated structures. Often these patients have not been thoroughly evaluated from a manual therapy standpoint and specific joint limitation, soft tissue immobility, and adverse mechanical neural tension are present that have hindered the rehabilitation process. Many times structure(s) at fault are not initially identified and, therefore, are not addressed with the exercise program. Manual therapists trained in the Australian approach firmly believe that if the complaint is reproducible, then it is likely that the complaint is treatable. Skillful manual palpation and assessment then resemble the physician's skillful use of the needle during many diagnostic tests.

The use of passive joint mobilization for cervical spine complaints is an integral aspect of the total cervical rehabilitation program. Highly trained manual therapists employ precise examination procedures to determine where passive joint mobilization fits in to the treatment program. Logical clinical decision-making skills and continual reassessment assist in selection of technique and a successful treatment outcome.

REFERENCES

1. Arnoldi CC, Reimann IM, Christensen SB, et al: The effect of joint position in juxtaarticular bone marrow pressure. Acta Orthop Scand 51:893–897, 1980.
2. Aspinalli W: Clinical testing for cervical mechanical disorders which produce ischemic vertigo. Orthop Sports Phys Ther 11:176–182, 1989.
3. Breig A: Adverse Mechanical Tension in the Central Nervous System. New York, John Wiley & Sons, 1978.
4. Bustrode C: Why are osteoarthritic joints painful? J Roy Naval Med Ser 62:5–16, 1976.
5. Butler D: Adverse mechanical tension in the nervous system: A mode for assessment and treatment. Aust J Physiotherapy 35:227–238, 1989.
6. Cloward R: Cervical diskography. Ann Surg 150:1052–1064, 1959.
7. Coman WB: Dizziness related to ENT conditions. In Grieve GP (ed): Modern Manual Therapy of the Vertebral Column. Edinburgh, Churchill Livingstone, 1986, pp 303–314.
8. Cyriax J: Textbook of Orthopaedic Medicine. London, Bailliere Tindall, 1974.
9. Edwards B: Combined movements in the cervical spine (C2–7); their value in examination and technique choice. Aust J Physiother 26:165–176, 1980.
10. Edwards BC: Combined movements of the cervical spine in examination and treatment. In Grant R (ed): Physical Therapy of the Cervical and Thoracic Spine. Edinburgh, Churchill Livingstone, 1988, pp 125–131.
11. Elvey RL: Brachial plexus tension tests and the pathoanatomical origin or arm pain. In Idczak RM (ed): Aspects of Manipulative Therapy. Carlton, Australia, Lincoln Institute of Health Sciences, 1981, pp 116–121.
12. Elvey R: The treatment of pain associated with abnormal brachial plexus tension. Aust J Physiotherapy 32:225–234, 1986.
13. Farrell J, Twomey L: Acute low back pain, comparison of two conservative treatment approaches. Med J Aust 1:160–164, 1982.
14. Feinstein B, Langston J, Jameson R, Schiller F: Experiments on pain referred from deep somatic tissues. J Bone Joint Surg 36A:981–997, 1954.
15. Ferrell W, Nade S, Newbold P: Inter-relation of neural discharge; intraarticular pressure, and joint angle in the knee of the dog. J Physiol 373:353–365, 1986.
16. Frank C, Akeson W, Woo S, et al: Physiology and therapeutic value of passive joint motion. Clin Orthop Rel Res 185:113–125, 1984.
17. Frykholm R: Cervical root compression resulting from disc degeneration and root sleeve fibrosis. Acta Chir Scand Suppl, 160, 1951.
18. Giovanelli-Blacker B, Elvey R, Thompson E: The clinical significance of measured lumbar zygoapophyseal intra-capsular pressure variation. In Proceedings of Manipulative Therapists Association of Australia. Brisbane, Australia, 1985.
19. Grant R: Dizziness testing and manipulation of the cervical spine. In Grant R (ed): Physical Therapy of the Cervical and Thoracic Spine. Edinburgh, Churchill Livingstone, 1988, pp 111–124.
20. Green D, Joynt R: Vascular accidents associated with neck manipulation. JAMA 170:522–528, 1959.
21. Grieve G: Common Vertebral Joint Problems. Edinburgh, Churchill Livingstone, 1981.

22. Grieve GP: Mobilization of the Spine. Notes on Examination, Assessment and Clinical Method, 4th ed. Edinburgh, Churchill Livingstone, 1984.
23. Jones LH: Strain and Counterstrain. Newark, OH, American Academy of Osteopathy, 1981.
24. Jull G, Bodguk N, Marsland A: The accuracy of manual diagnosis for cervical zygoapophyseal joint pain syndromes. Med J Aust 148:233–236, 1988.
25. Kaltenborn F: Mobilisation I. Sementi mobilis columna vertebalis. Oslo, Norway Byadoy, 1975.
26. Kellgren J: Observations on referred pain arising from muscle. Clin Sci 3:175–193, 1938.
27. Kellgren J: On the distribution of pain arising from deep somatic structures with charts of segmental pain areas. Clin Sci 4:35–46, 1939.
28. Kenneally M, Rubenach H, Elvey R: The upper limb tension test: The SLR test of the arm. In Grant R (ed): Physical Therapy of the Cervical and Thoracic Spine. Edinburgh, Churchill Livingstone, 1988, pp 167–194.
29. Korr IM: Neurochemical and neurotrophic consequences of nerve deformation. In Glasgow EF, Twomey LT, Skull ER, et al (eds): Aspects of Manipulative Therapy. Melbourne, Churchill Livingstone, 1985, pp 64–71.
30. Kvist M, Jarvenen M: Clinical, histochemical and biochemical features in repair of muscle and tension injuries. Int J Sports Med 3:12–14, 1982.
31. Levick J: An investigation into the validity of subatmospheric pressure recordings from synovial fluid and their dependence on joint angle. J Physiol 289:55–67, 1979.
32. MacKinnon J: Osteoporosis: A review. Phys Ther 68:1533–1539, 1988.
33. Magarey ME: Examination and assessment of spinal joint dysfunction. In Greive GP (ed): Modern Manual Therapy of the Vertebral Column. Edinburgh, Churchill Livingstone, 1986, pp 481–497.
34. Maitland G: Negative disc exploration, positive canal signs. Aust J Physiotherapy 25:129–134, 1979.
35. Maitland G: Palpation examination of the posterior cervical spine: Ideal, average, and normal. Aust J Physiotherapy 28:3–12, 1982.
36. Maitland GD: Vertebral Manipulation, 5th ed. London, Butterworth. 1986.
37. McKenzie R: The Lumbar Spine: Mechanical Diagnosis and Therapy. Waikanae, New Zealand, Spinal Publ Ltd., 1981.
38. Mennel J: Back Pain. Boston, Little, Brown, 1960.
39. Mitchell FL, Moran PS, Pruzzo NA: An Evaluation and Treatment Manual of Osteopathetic Muscle Energy Procedures, Part III. Published by authors. P.O. Box 371, Valley Park, MO 63088 USA, 1979.
40. Overton L: Cervical spine nerve root pain. Am Surg 17:343, 1951.
41. Paris S: Mobilization of the spine. Phys Ther 59:988–995, 1979.
42. Parker G, Tupling H, Pryor D: A controlled trial of cervical manipulation for migraine. Aust NZ J Med 8:589–593, 1978.
43. Reynolds M: Myofascial trigger point syndromes in the practice of rheumatology. Arch Phys Med Rehabil 62:111–113, 1981.
44. Schellhas K, Latchow R, Wendling L, et al: Vertebrobasilar injuries following cervical manipulation. JAMA 244:145, 1980.
45. Simeone FA, Rothman RH: Cervical disc disease. In Rothman RH, Simeone FA (eds): The Spine, Vol. 1. Philadelphia, W.B. Saunders, 1975, p 387.
46. Sloop P, Smith D, Goldberg E, Dore C: Manipulation for chronic neck pain, a double blind study. Spine 7:532–533, 1982.
47. Stevens BJ, McKenzie RA: Mechanical diagnosis and self treatment of the cervical spine. In Grant R (ed): Physical Therapy of the Cervical and Thoracic Spine, Edinburgh, Churchill Livingstone, 1988, pp 271–289.
48. Trott PH: Manipulative therapy techniques in the management of some cervical syndromes. In Grant R (ed): Physical Therapy of the Cervical and Thoracic Spine. Edinburgh, Churchill Livingstone, 1988, pp 219–241.
49. Ward R: Headache: An osteopathic perspective. J Am Osteopathic Assoc 81:458–466, 1982.
50. Wilkinson M (ed): Cervical Spondylosis, 2nd ed. London, Heineman, 1971.
51. Woo S, Gomez M, Amiel D, et al: The effects of exercise on the biomechanical and biochemical properties of swine digital flexor tendon. J Biomech Eng 103:51–56, 1981.
52. Wright V, Dawson N: Biomechanics of joint function. In Holt PLJ (ed): Current Topics in Connective Tissue Disease. Edinburgh, Churchill Livingstone, 1975, p 115.
53. Wyke B, Polacek P: Articular neurology: The present position. J Bone Joint Surg 57B:401, 1975.

TARA SWEENEY, PT
CAROL PRENTICE
JEFFREY A. SAAL, MD
JOEL S. SAAL, MD

CERVICOTHORACIC MUSCULAR STABILIZATION TECHNIQUES

Tara Sweeney, PT
Carol Prentice,
    Alexander Technique Trainer
Jeffrey A. Saal, MD,
    Director, Research & Education
Joel S. Saal, MD,
    Physiatrist
San Francisco Spine Institute
Daly City, California

Reprint requests to:
San Francisco Spine Institute
1850 Sullivan Avenue
Suite 140
Daly City, CA 94015

This chapter introduces the concept and basis of cervicothoracic stabilization training (CTST). Traditionally, the patient with cervicothoracic pain has been treated with cervical collars, cervical traction, ultrasound, electric stimulation, soft tissue massage, and joint mobilization.[1,8] Although these techniques may form an integral part of the early treatment process, they also rely more heavily on the practitioner than on active patient participation.

Rehabilitation of the cervicothoracic spine patient requires a comprehensive approach. To be successful, a program must include active patient participation. The program should teach the patient to assume control of his or her cervicothoracic condition. The primary goals of the CTST program are to maximize return to function, to limit progression of degenerative changes, and to prevent further injury. Functional improvement gives the patient realistic goals and expectations as well as an objective outcome. The overall rehabilitation program should be designed to accommodate the individual's needs, lifestyle, available training time, and occupation.

ASSESSMENT OF PHYSICAL AND FUNCTIONAL CAPACITY

Prior to the commencement of the training program, accurate assessments of the patient's physical and functional capacity are required. An accurate diagnosis and complete functional examination provide the guidelines for program progression.[11] Localization and clinical reproduction of symptoms in specific posture patterns are essential to designing the initial training program. Consistent reproduction of symptoms with postural positioning and relief through posture alteration are key to identifying the initial functional range. The determinants of functional range often encompass variable factors such as the underlying pathologic condition and secondary bony restrictions, muscular restrictions, irregularity of force coupling patterns of movement, and inflammation. Therefore, careful correlation of the patient's history, mechanism of injury, and physical and functional examinations is important in recognizing abnormal movement patterns.

The cervical spine must permit support of the head while allowing great degrees of movement to optimize function of the sensory organs housed within the cranium. Cervical spine mobility should allow an individual to look quickly behind, over the shoulders, up at the stars, and down at a newspaper. The cervical spine moves in flexion, extension, lateral flexion, and rotation. Lateral flexion and rotation are considered to be combined movements.[2,4,6]

Total movement of the cervical spine is the composite of segmental motion of all the cervical vertebrae. The major portion of rotational movement occurs in the upper cervical portion between the occiput, the atlas, and the axis.[2] The remaining motion occurs at the lower cervical segments C4–C7.[2]

Poor posture and irregular movement patterns alter the normal segmental use of cervical vertebrae. Postures considered poor or undesirable are those that aggravate dorsal thoracic kyphosis, resulting in rounding of the shoulders. Faulty posture thrusts the head forward from the lower cervical spine and increases upper cervical lordosis with compensatory occipital-atlas extension (Fig. 1).[3,8]

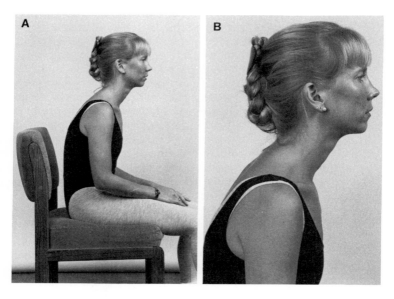

FIGURE 1. *A*, Increase in thoracic kyphosis associated with scapular protraction and a reversion of the lumbar lordosis. *B*, Leading chin position and exaggeration of cervical lordosis.

Poor posture during lifting, carrying, pushing, and pulling may contribute to forward translation and compression stresses on cervical structures.

Movement patterns on a poor postural base contribute to repetitive microtrauma of cervical structures, including facets, discs, ligaments, articular capsules, and muscles. These patterns of movement contribute to habitual overuse of isolated motion segments while they minimize normal movement at others. Habitual dysfunction of isolated segments may generate bony hypertrophy, ligamentous laxity, and breakdown of disc and facet articulations.[11] The underlying combination can perpetuate itself in pain, spasm, and the dysfunction cycle.[9,11]

Correct dispersal of segmental movement depends on the balanced relationship between the head (occiput), the cervical spine, and the thoracic cage. This balanced relationship is termed the position of optimal function (POF) (Fig. 2). POF is the functional range of the cervical spine in which each segment operates in its safest, most balanced, and pain-free position. It is a position that optimizes the biomechanical balance between the thoracic "base" and the flexible, balanced cervical spine. POF does not mean eliminating all lordosis by forcing a dorsal glide into a military posture. Rather POF is a balanced position with slight occipital-atlas flexion and the comfortable or small degree of cervical lordosis available to each individual.

Alteration of this cervical position may not be attempted without consideration of the entire spine. All spinal curves transect a plumb line to remain in balance with gravity (Fig. 3).[2] An increase in any one curve must be compensated for by a proportionate increase or decrease in the other curves (Fig. 4). For example, lumbar flexion associated with slump sitting contributes to collapse of the thoracic cage or increased thoracic kyphosis. The increased thoracic kyphosis and rounded shoulders provide a poor base of support for the cervical spine. This poor base thrusts the head forward at the cervicothoracic junction with resultant compensatory occipital-atlas extension position.

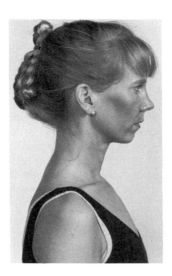

FIGURE 2.   Chin-down position coupled with scapular retraction.

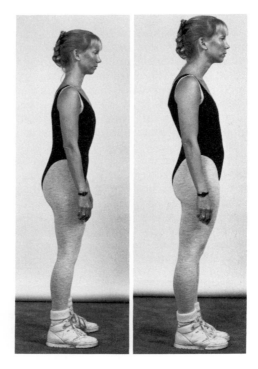

FIGURE 3 *(left).*   Balanced lumbar posture leading to a balanced cervicothoracic curve.

FIGURE 4 *(right).*   Increase in lumbar lordosis will necessitate a second counterbalancing of increase in thoracic kyphosis, finally leading to cervical lordosis in the "chin forward, stooped shoulders" position.

STABILIZATION OF THE LUMBAR SPINE

Training the balanced cervical spine must, therefore, include postural stabilization retraining of the entire spine. Lumbar spine stabilization offers a properly aligned base of support for the thoracic cage. If the thoracic cage is conceptualized as the platform upon which the cervical spine rests, the thoracic cage position is the key to postural control of the balanced cervical spine.

The critical components of a balanced spine are muscular strength and symmetry. The anterior and posterior muscles of the thoracic cage may be thought of as cables that effectively influence the articular interaction of the thoracic spine, scapulothoracic articulation, and glenohumeral joints.

Shortening of the anterior musculature, including the pectoralis major, pectoralis minor, and anterior deltoid muscles, contributes to a shortened, narrow, and collapsed thoracic cage. Pectoralis minor muscle fibers run inferiorly, obliquely, and medially, forming the tip of the coracoid process to the anterior third through fifth rib. The fibers pull the anteroscapulae laterally and anteriorly, resulting in rounded shoulders.

A lengthened, widened, and opened thoracic cage requires equivalent soft tissue extensibility between these muscle groups. Additionally, the posterior interscapular musculature, including the middle and lower fibers of the trapezius, rhomboid, and serratus anterior muscles, must be both flexible and strong enough to support the "shoulders back, chest out" posture.

The muscles with force vectors that lie anteriorly and posteriorly to the cervical spine also act as cables that influence the joint alignment and symmetry of the head and cervical spine in relation to the thoracic cage. A shortening of the suboccipital, sternocleidomastoid, upper trapezius, levator scapulae, splenius capitis, longissimus capitis, spinalis capitis, and semispinalis capitis musculature contributes to a flattened lower cervical spine with a compensatory occiput-atlas extension position (Table 1). Lengthening of these muscles in balance with the anterior flexors frees up the motion segments to attain a balanced position of the occiput resting upon the atlas. The balanced neutral cervical position offers an appropriate starting base for segmental mobility and stabilization training.

The stability of the cervical column depends upon dynamic muscular control. The musculature must be strong and symmetric for position maintenance during cervicothoracic training. This will reduce compression forces, chronic soft tissue strain, and excessive forces upon the cervical intervertebral discs.

STABILIZATION TRAINING

CTST requires specialized training and coordination in the use of body mechanics, posture, movement principles, and active exercise. The principles of stabilization training include retraining the musculature to control and use cervical mobility and stability of the diseased (painful) spinal segment. CTST promotes the necessary strength, coordination, and endurance to maintain the cervical spine in a stable and safe position during loading, mobility, and weight-bearing activities. Stabilization training optimizes the capacity of the cervicothoracic spine to absorb loads in all directions while it maintains minimizes direct stress and strain on individual cervical tissues. It eliminates repetitive microtrauma to the cervical segments and limits progression of injury, allowing healing to take place.[11]

Cervicothoracic stabilization training focuses on balance of the neutral spine, restoration of segmental mobility, dynamic muscular control, and the appropriate use of stabilization principles. The components of training must, therefore, encompass mobility as well as stability within a functional range.

TABLE 1. Soft Tissue Flexibility Training: Major Areas of Concern

Anterior Muscles	Posterior Muscles
Sternocleidomastoid	Rectus capitis posterior major
Scaleni	Rectus capitis posterior minor
Pectoralis major	Obliquus capitis inferior
Pectoralis minor	Obliquus capitis superior
Biceps (long head)	Levator scapulae
	Superior trapezius
	Latissimus dorsi
	Teres major
	Subscapularis
	Rhomboids
	Middle trapezius
	Lower trapezius
	Serratus anterior

Mobility

The emphasis of the mobility phase is restoration of segmental movement from a balanced position. It is important to enhance dynamic stability while avoiding cervical joint fixation and soft tissue rigidity. Additionally, restoration of motion may be limited by pain and pathologic changes.[10] A fine line exists between a tolerable range of movement and the end range; at the end range the patient's symptoms will be exacerbated. Proper flexibility and mobility exercises applied to the area of restriction give the patient a valuable tool for controlling pain and improving function.[10] Flexibility training geared at restoring lost movement is discussed later in the chapter.

Stability

While mobility provides an important function in daily living, stabilization in the balanced position is essential when lifting, carrying, pushing, and pulling objects. Muscle control helps to maintain the balanced position during performance of daily tasks using the upper and lower extremities independent of the trunk/spine. Spinal stabilization training focuses on co-contraction of axial musculature while allowing isolated movement at the peripheral joints.

Dynamic stabilization involves a large range of muscular activity, depending on the task. For example, an activity such as backing a car out of a driveway requires mobility in conjunction with contraction of muscles to place the head in a position to increase the visual field.

An activity such as lifting an object requires muscular stabilization of the cervical spine in a safe position while the forces are transmitted away from the spine to the upper and lower extremities. Cervicothoracic training must encompass the range from mobility to stability by altering the type of exercise, the position of exercise, the resistance of exercise, and related functional activities.

Initial Patient Education

During an acute phase of pain, rest of the injured areas and use of cervical supports may be indicated. The cervical supports should hold the neck in a comfortable, balanced position. Initial patient education entails neck first aid, positions of comfort, time-contingent activity and rest, application of ice, and body mechanics. The patient learns hands-on control of symptoms that may occur while performing activities of daily living.

The training phase begins with the patient's education in "neck and back basics." The purpose of "back basics" is to instruct the patient with either a low back or cervical thoracic injury about the basic concepts of spine care, spinal anatomy, the neutral spine, and stabilization.

Postural Reeducation

Following neck and back basics, postural reeducation begins. A balanced posture is the "state of muscular and skeletal balance that protects supporting structures of the body against injury or progressive deformity regardless of the attitude."[2]

The cervical spine is a very flexible structure that can be tilted, rotated, and lowered by contracting the muscles attached to it. Balanced on top of the cervical spine is the head with its center of gravity anterior to its base, the atlas.[2] The ligaments and muscles of the neck, with their insertion points at the base of the skull, play a key role in maintaining a balanced position of the head in relationship to the cervical and thoracic spine (see Figs. 2 and 3).[2]

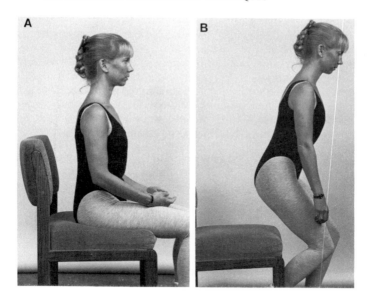

FIGURE 5. *A*, Reduction of thoracic kyphosis and associated flattening of the cervical spine. *B*, Transition position: note the lack of cervical extension that should correctly accompany position transition, as opposed to an extension synergy pattern.

The therapist begins by having the patient sit with front and side mirror views. This positioning enables the patient to see any postural deviations of the spine. It is important for the patient to see his or her habitual posture in order to facilitate change (Fig. 5).

Next, the therapist helps the patient to find a neutral balanced position of the lumbar and cervicothoracic spine. Instruction includes verbal and subtle hands-on cuing. With the patient's feet on the floor in front of him, the patient sits balanced upon the ischial tuberosities in a stabilized lumbar spine position. The therapist then demonstrates to the patient the neutral position of the thoracic cage and cervical spine in relationship to the lumbar spine. Generally, this involves lengthening the anterior and posterior soft tissues with special attention to releasing the posterior neck muscles, thereby allowing the head to assume a slightly forward and balanced position upon the cervical spine. If the patient's condition is acute, this training may need to begin in the supine position.

The next phase of postural reeducation is to use the balanced neutral position in a basic movement sequence such as a transition from sitting to standing. In this sequence the patient has a tendency to extend the head back and down, as well as tighten the posterior and posterolateral muscles of the neck. The therapist instructs and directs the patient to move forward from the hips while maintaining a neutral spine and allowing the chin to drop slightly while leaving the chair (see Fig. 5). Most patients will not realize that they are pulling their heads back and tightening their neck muscles in this habitual movement pattern. A hand on the back of the neck helps to demonstrate this pattern and provides kinesthetic feedback.

Flexibility

If the patient is unable to attain a balanced cervical position because of soft tissue or joint restrictions, the next step must include flexibility training before proceeding. Flexibility is an integral component of cervicothoracic stabilization training. Adequate flexibility of the anterior chest wall, interscapular region, and cervical musculature is necessary in order to assume a balanced posture.

Isolation of upper extremity movement without compensatory cervicothoracic motion requires adequate flexibility of the shoulder girdle musculature, especially the internal rotators. Additionally, restoration of normal scapulothoracic movement must be accomplished.[8,9]

The two components of cervical flexibility are **joint mobility** and **soft tissue extensibility**. Joint mobility is accomplished through mobilization techniques.

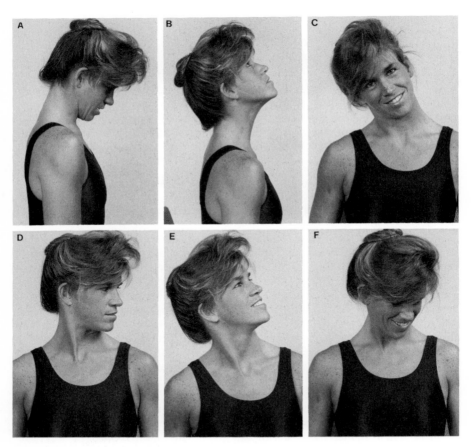

FIGURE 6. *A,* Forward flexion stretching the posterior soft tissues. *B,* Extension stretching the anterior soft tissues. *C,* Lateral flexion principally stretching the contralateral upper trapezius. *D,* Cervical rotation stretching a combination of posterior lateral and anterior tissues. *E,* Combined extension-rotation principally stretching contralateral, deep, anterior soft tissues. *F,* Combined flexion-rotation principally stretching contralateral, upper lateral soft tissues.

Mobilization describes the application of a force along the rotational or translational planes of motion of a joint.[12] Specific joint mobilization may be accomplished through a gentle, active range-of-motion exercise as demonstrated in Figure 6. Clearly defined beginning and ending positions with careful attention to movement of the segment in question are essential to correct execution of the exercise. An appropriate exercise applied improperly does not achieve the desired effect.[10]

Stretching techniques provide increased soft tissue extensibility. Stretching defines an activity that applies a deforming force along a linear plane of motion.[12] The shortened musculature in the cervical, scapulothoracic, and shoulder girdle areas is the chief targets for stretching (see Table 1). The specific muscle groups are categorized as anterior or posterior. The anterior muscle groups include the sternocleidomastoid, scaleni, pectoralis major, pectoralis minor, and the long head of the bicep. The posterior muscle groups are the deep occipital muscles, i.e., rectus capitis posterior major and minor, obliquus capitis inferior and superior, levator scapulae, superior trapezius, latissimus dorsi, teres major, subscapularis, tricep, and posterior deltoid.

Techniques proved to be effective in promoting musculotendinous flexibility include ballistic stretching, passive stretching, static stretching, and neuromuscular facilitation. Ballistic stretching is not recommended, because repeated bouncing stretches the contracting muscle and may lead to further injury. Early passive stretching by the treating practitioner should be performed with caution. A sustained stretch beyond the patient's safe available excursion may prolong symptoms or cause additional injury. It is advisable to instruct the patient to initiate static stretching at the middle or end of the tolerable range of motion. Static stretching requires spine safe techniques. The stretch is initiated from the balanced position. Prevention of collapsed thoracic cage and forward head positioning minimizes abnormal stretching patterns. A position that applies a gradual stretch to the cervical musculature (Fig. 7) and upper extremity musculature (Fig. 8) is achieved and maintained for a 15–60 second period.

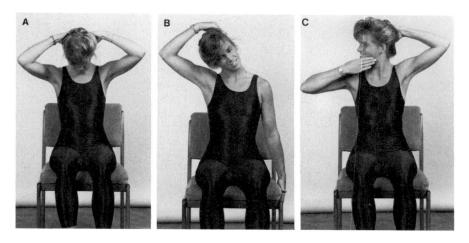

FIGURE 7. *A,* Position neck stretch. *B,* Cervical lateral flexion stretch. *C,* Cervical rotational stretch.

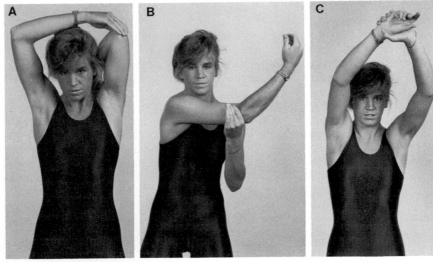

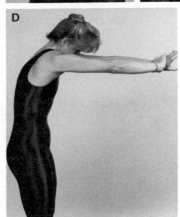

FIGURE 8. *A,* Triceps and interior shoulder capsule stretch. *B,* Posterior deltoid and posterior shoulder capsule stretch. *C,* Latissimus dorsi and teres major stretch. *D,* Interscapular/rhomboid stretch.

An improved range of shortened soft tissue musculature restores capacity for normal movement patterns. Full range is desired for tissue health and function. It minimizes and/or prevents abnormal excursion, which contributes to adaptive shortening and functional disability. Finally, it establishes adequate extensibility of tissues for dynamic stability versus protective rigid stability.

It is important to stabilize the shoulder girdle prior to stretching the cervical musculature. This stabilization may be accomplished by grabbing the base of a chair (demonstrated in Figure 7B) to depress and stabilize the shoulder girdle, and to prevent it from moving. Once the shoulder girdle is stabilized, the head is directed away from the shoulder in rotation, lateral flexion, or combined patterns. As the available excursion improves, a steady application of additional force may be added by the use of proper hand placement. If deficits in range of motion remain after patient instruction, then passive stretching and neuromuscular facilitation techniques are appropriate. These methods require a skilled practitioner to perform hold-relax and contract-relax methods to the appropriate shortened musculature.

As normal range of both joint and soft tissue is achieved, muscle strength, endurance, and coordination may be addressed through stabilization routines.

The Lumbar Stabilization Exercise Program

The good cervicothoracic program begins with a lumbar stabilization program. Lumbar stabilization programs include exercises such as partial sit-ups, diagonal sit-ups, prone reciprocal arm and leg, and superman. Necessary precautions in monitoring and supporting the spine during this initial phase are important so as not to exacerbate cervical symptoms. The lumbar stabilization exercise program strengthens and aligns the lumbopelvic base of support for a neutral cervicothoracic posture (Table 2).

TABLE 2. The Progression of Cervicothoracic Stabilization Exercises

	Cervicothoracic Stabilization Levels		
	I Basic	II Intermediate	III Advanced
Direct Cervical Stabilization Exercises	Cervical active range of motion Cervical isometrics	Cervical gravity Resisted isometrics	Cervical active Range gravity resisted
Indirect Cervical Stabilization Exercises			
Supine, head supported	Theraband chest press Bilateral arm raise Supported dying bug	Unsupported dying bug	Chest flyes Bench press Incline dumbbell press
Sit	Reciprocal arm raise Unilateral arm raise Bilateral arm raise Seated row Latissimus pulldown	Swiss ball reciprocal Arm raises Chest press	Swiss ball bilateral Shoulder shrugs Supraspinatus raises

Stand	Theraband reciprocal
	Chest press
	Theraband straight
	Arm latissimus
	Pulldown
	Theraband:
	  Chest press
	  Latissimus pulldown
	Standing rowing
	Crossovers
	Tricep press
		Standing rowing
		Bicep pulldown
			Upright row
			Shoulder shrugs
			Supraspinatus raises

Flexed hip-hinge position	0–30° Reciprocal arm raise Unilateral arm raise Bilateral arm raise Interscapular flyes	30–60° Incline prone flyes Reciprocal deltoid raise Cable crossovers	60–90° Bilateral anterior Deltoid raises Interscapular flyes
Prone	Reciprocal arm raise Unilateral arm raise Bilateral arm raise	Quadruped Head unsupported Swiss ball bilateral Anterior deltoid raises Swiss ball prone Rowing Swiss ball prone flyes	Head supported Prone flyes Latissimus flyes
Supine, head unsupported	Not advised for Level I	Partial sit-ups Arm raises	Swiss ball chest flyes Swiss ball reciprocal

Treatment Phases

A. Stabilization Program
 1. Finding Neutral Position
    a. Standing
    b. Sitting
    c. Jumping
    d. Prone
 2. Prone Gluteal Squeezes
    a. With arm raises
    b. With alternate arm
       raises
    c. With leg raises
    d. With alternate leg raises
    e. With arm and leg raises
    f. With alternate arm and
       leg raises
 3. Supine Pelvic Bracing
 4. Bridging Progression
    a. Basic position
    b. One leg raised
    c. With ankle weights stepping
    d. With ankle weights balanced
       on gym ball
 5. Quadruped
    a. With alternating arm and
       leg movements
    b. With ankle and wrist weights

 6. Kneeling Stabilization
    a. Double knee
    b. Single knee
    c. Lunges
       1. Without weight
       2. With weight
 7. Wall Slide Quadriceps Strengthening
 8. Position Transition with Postural Control
    a. Abdominal program
       1. Curl-ups
       2. Dying bug
          a. Supported
          b. Unsupported
       3. Diagonal curl-ups
       4. Diagonal curl-ups on incline
          board
       5. Straight leg lowering
    b. Gym program
       1. Latissimus pulldowns
       2. Angled leg press
       3. Lunges
       4. Hyperextension bench
       5. General upper weight exercises
       6. Pulley exercises to stress postural
          control

Regional Exercises

Cervicothoracic stabilization training may be divided into regional exercises for the cervical, interscapular, chest, and upper extremity musculature. The patient must learn to use muscle groups in an isolated fashion as well as in co-contraction patterns, performing increasingly difficult tasks and putting increased demands on the body.

The regional musculature of the cervical spine includes cervical spinal extensors and anterior musculature, i.e., rectus capitis anterior, rectus capitis lateralis, longissimus cervicis, and longus capitis. The anterior musculature stabilizes the cervical spine in the neutral position during muscular contraction of the sternocleidomastoid, as when raising a patient's head off the table while in the supine position (see Fig. 10C). Emphasis is placed on the cervical extensors to balance shear stress on the intervertebral segments.

The primary thoracic stabilizers are the abdominal, spinal extensor, and latissimus dorsi muscles. In the scapulothoracic area, the major muscles of concern include the middle and lower trapezius, serratus anterior, and rhomboids. The chest wall muscles to concentrate on include the clavicular head of the pectoralis major and pectoralis minor. The upper extremity muscles—supraspinatus, bicep, tricep, and deltoid—also require training.

Exercise Progression

As the program advances, the patient is instructed in co-contraction techniques that consist of active use of the trunk-stabilizing muscles to balance the spine while an extremity performs a task. Advancing the type, position, and resistance of the exercise provides a progression of cervicothoracic stabilization

TABLE 3.   Variables for Cervicothoracic Stabilization Progression

Training Level	Trunk Position	Exercise Pattern	Resistance Type
I Basic	Supine Sit Kneel Stand Flexed hip-hinge position (0–30°)* Prone	(a) Reciprocal arm movement (b) Unilateral arm movement	Theraband (elastic resistance)
II Intermediate	Supine Sit Kneel Stand Flexed hip-hinge position (30–60°)* Prone Transition positions: •Sit-stand •Supine-sit	(a) Reciprocal arm movement (b) Unilateral arm movement	(a) Weight machine (b) Pulleys (c) Free weights
III Advanced	Supine Sit Kneel Stand Flexed hip-hinge position (60–90°)* Prone Balanced challenge: Swiss ball Transition positions: •Sit-stand •Supine-sit	(a) Reciprocal arm movement (b) Unilateral arm movement (c) Bilateral arm movement (d) Predictable loading[†]	(a) Weight machine (b) Pulleys (c) Free weights (d) Free form objects
IV Advanced Athlete	Free form	(a) Specialized sports drills[†] (b) Unexpected loading[‡] (c) Falls (d) Contact (football tackling and blocking) (e) Power drills[§]	Live sports activity

* See Figure 17.
[†] Tasks that involve cervicothoracic load placement accomplished in definable postural positions, e.g., lifting a box from a high shelf.
[‡] Loads placed upon the cervicothoracic spine that occur without warning and in various postural positions, e.g., catching a falling object or bracing for a sudden fall.
[§] High-speed movement patterns using near maximal loads.

training. Cervicothoracic exercises presented here are arranged according to these principles of program progression (Table 3). The types of exercise selected challenge the individual's stabilization skills by altering the activity from static positioning to dynamic balancing. Each exercise incorporates varying degrees of upper extremity movement, progressing from unilateral arm raises, to reciprocal arm raises, to bilateral arm raises. The patient's stabilization skills may continue to be challenged with transitional movements. Transitional movements include a change of position such as sitting to standing or entire body movement in space such as pivoting and turning. The movement from the supine position to the sitting position may be a difficult stabilization skill for the patient to achieve.

Once stabilization skills are mastered in the transitional movement phase of the program, predictable loading and unexpected loading may be added. The patient's balance may be challenged with the use of the Swiss gymnastic ball. Power drills involving speed, strength, falls, and contact require the highest level of stabilization skills.

Exercise Position

Varying exercise position determines the required amount of trunk stabilization. Initially, exercises can be performed in the supine position with the head supported in the balanced position. Exercises progress to the sitting, kneeling, and standing positions. Finally, the prone and the flexed hinge-hip stance positions may be introduced into the program. The flexed hinge-hip stance is a standing position with varying degrees of knee and hip flexion (see Fig. 17).

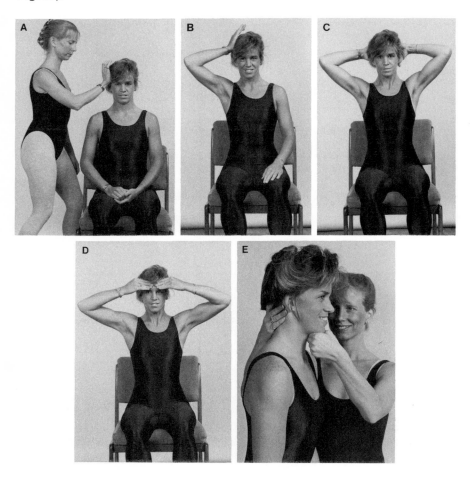

FIGURE 9. *A,* Isometric lateral flexion. *B,* Isometric lateral flexion. *C,* Isometric extension. *D,* Isometric forward flexion. *E,* Isometric upper cervical flexion.

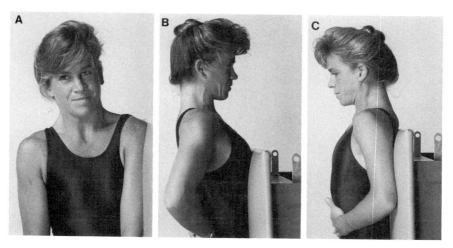

FIGURE 10. *A,* Gravity resisted: isometric lateral flexion. *B,* Gravity resisted: isometric extension. *C,* Gravity resisted: isometric forward flexion.

Resistance Exercises

The type of resistance advances from isometric to isotonic contractions. During isometric contractions, the muscle remains at a constant length. Isometrics vary the patient's positioning and direction relative to gravity, resulting in direct stabilization of the cervical spine. Initially, the patient may begin isometrics in the supine position with the head supported, and then progresses to isometrics in the seated position (Fig. 9) or off the edge of a table against gravity (Fig. 10). Exercises are performed with the cervical spine in the neutral position. An active range of resistance results in dynamic stabilization of the cervical spine (Figs. 11 and 12).

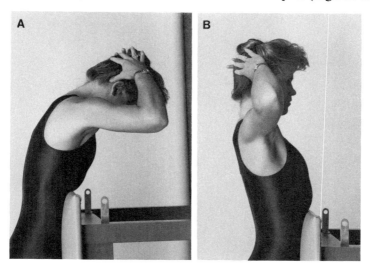

FIGURE 11. *A,* Initial position: active gravity-resisted cervicothoracic extension position. *B,* Final position: active gravity-resisted cervicothoracic extension.

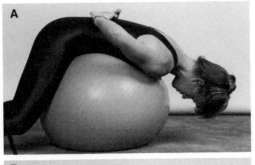

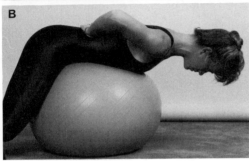

FIGURE 12. *A,* Initial position: Swiss ball, active, gravity-resisted cervicothoracic extension start position. *B,* Final position: Swiss ball, active, gravity-resisted cervicothoracic extension.

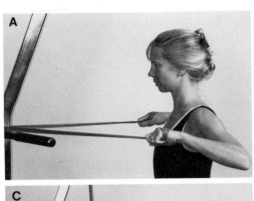

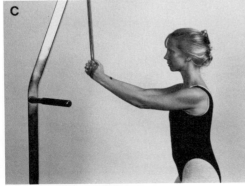

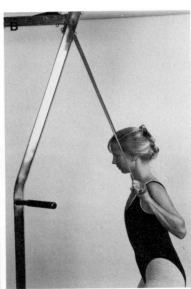

FIGURE 13. *A,* Theraband resisted rowing while standing. *B,* Theraband resisted rowing while pulldown. *C,* Theraband resisted pulldown.

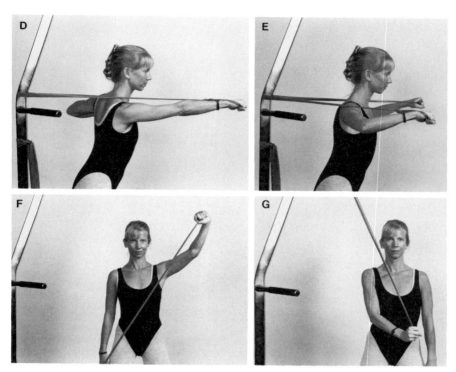

FIGURE 13 *(Continued)*. *D*, Theraband resisted reciprocal chest press. *E*, Theraband resisted chest press while standing. *F*, Theraband resisted diagonal external rotation. *G*, Theraband resisted diagonal internal rotation.

Dynamic cervical stabilization requires great segmental control from a neutral spine position. It is restricted to the tolerable range available to each patient. Avoidance of end range movement can minimize the exacerbation of symptoms.

Training the interscapular, shoulder, and upper extremity musculature provides indirect stabilization support for the cervical muscles. The training must couple co-contraction of cervicothoracic stabilizers with isotonic contractions of interscapular, shoulder, and upper extremity musculature against resistance. Methods of resistance during isotonic contractions progress from rubber tubing or Theraband (Figs. 13 and 14) to pulley systems (Fig. 15) and free weights (Figs. 16 to 20), and, finally, free body weight such as boxes. Rubber tubing, Theraband, a Swiss gym ball, and 3- to 6-pound dumbbells can provide the diversity necessary for a successful home program.

Prior to gym training, the patient must demonstrate consistent postural control and stabilization skill. Gym training challenges the stabilization ability of the patient; therefore, skill level assessment is necessary prior to advancement. The training goals include increasing muscular strength and endurance of trunk-stabilizing and extremity musculature in a spine safe technique. Targeted exercises for the shoulder girdle are listed in Table 4. Targeted exercises for the upper trunk or interscapular region are listed in Table 5. Table 6 provides the targeted groups for the upper extremity.

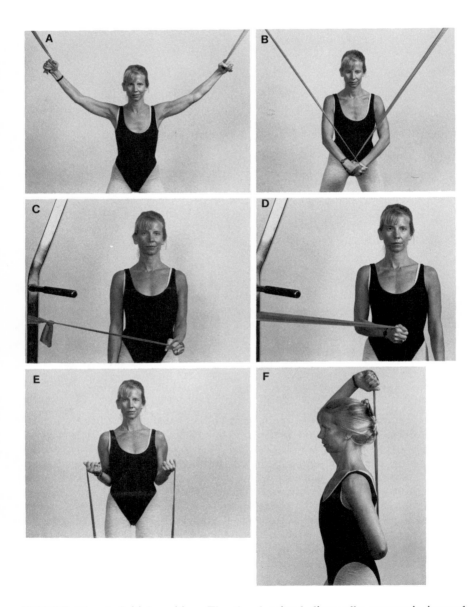

FIGURE 14. *A*, Initial position: Theraband-resisted diagonally symmetric internal rotation. *B*, Final position: Theraband-resisted diagonally symmetric internal rotation. *C*, Theraband-resisted external rotation pulls. *D*, Theraband-resisted internal rotation pulls. *E*, Theraband-resisted biceps curl in standing position. *F*, Theraband-resisted triceps curl in standing position.

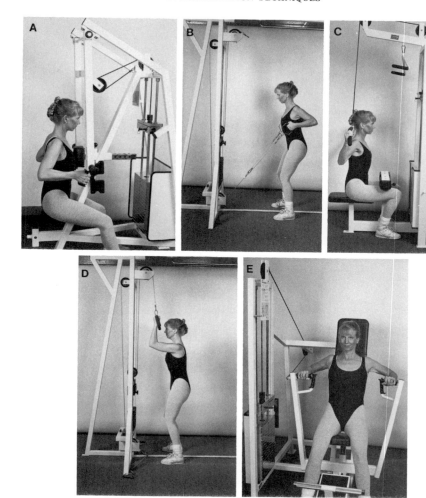

FIGURE 15.   *A,* Seated rowing. *B,* Rowing from a low pulley while standing. *C,* Closed hand pulldown. *D,* Open hand pulldown. *E,* Chest press.

Resistance exercises build additional strength, power, and endurance. The type of resistance, number of sets, and repetitions determine whether strength, power, or endurance will be trained. Specificity of training with sets and repetitions must match the individual's activities of daily living, occupation, and sports.

Exercises always must be matched with the patient's strength, endurance, and stabilization ability. Pain is one guide for exercise progression. An increase in axial or radicular pain requires reevaluation of the exercise program. An increase in pain may be caused by poor technique or inadequate coordination of available strength and endurance. Additionally, the pathologic condition may present a limitation to progression in the exercise program.

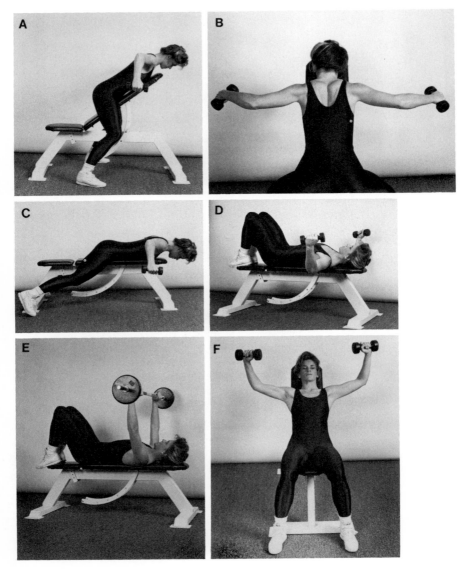

FIGURE 16. *A,* Incline prone flyes final position. *B,* Incline prone flyes posterior view. *C,* Prone flyes. *D,* Chest flyes. *E,* Bench press. *F,* Incline dumbbell press.

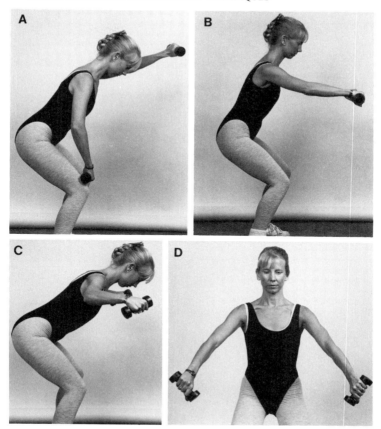

FIGURE 17. *A,* Flexed hinge-hip position reciprocal arm raise. *B,* Flexed hinge-hip position: anterior deltoid raises. *C,* Flexed hip-hinge position: reverse flyes (interscapular flyes). *D,* Supraspinatus raises in standing position.

CONCLUSION

Cervicothoracic stabilization training is a specialized program that requires coordination of body mechanics, posture, movement, posture, movement principles, and exercise to optimize spine function. It requires the balance of neutral spine, restoration of segmental mobility, and the appropriate use of stabilization principles. Stabilization training optimizes the capacity of the cervicothoracic spine to absorb loads in all directions while it minimizes direct stress and strain on individual cervical tissues.

When the patient becomes actively involved in the rehabilitation process, carryover and consistency of the stabilization training occur. The patient learns independence through self-management of symptoms and progression in the home program. The patient's heightened awareness of aggravating factors and the newly acquired ability to manage them with relieving positions, proper body mechanics, problem solving and favorable ergonomic design improves the patient's overall function. Training thus helps to control costs by reducing treatment time and limiting recidivism.

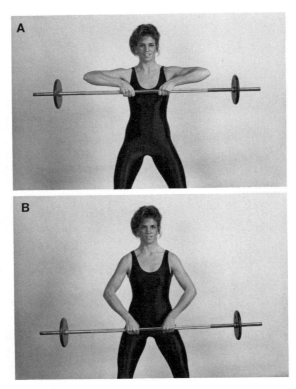

FIGURE 18. *A,* Initial position: upright rowing. *B,* Final position: upright rowing.

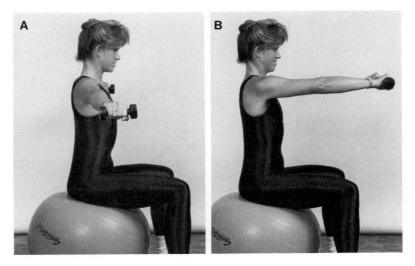

FIGURE 19. *A,* Lateral deltoid raises while seated on a Swiss gym ball. *B,* Anterior deltoid raises while seated on a Swiss gym ball.

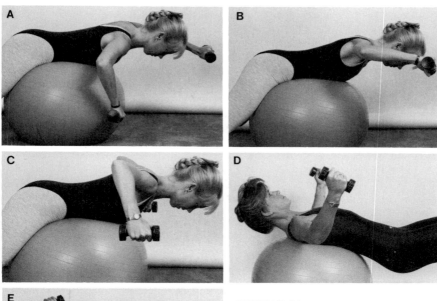

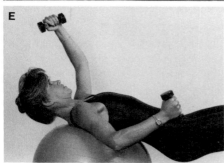

FIGURE 20.   *A*, Prone reciprocal arm raise while on a Swiss gym ball. *B*, Bilateral arm raises while on a Swiss gym ball. *C*, Prone flyes while on a Swiss gym ball. *D*, Chest flyes while on a Swiss gym ball. *E*, Supine reciprocal arm raises while on a Swiss gym ball.

TABLE 4.   Shoulder Girdle Muscle Strengthening Exercises Useful in Cervicothoracic Stabilization Training*

Exercise Routines	Figures	Primary Muscle Groups
Theraband resisted reciprocal chest press	Figure 13D	
Theraband resisted chest press while standing	Figure 13E	→ Pectoralis major
Initial and final positions: Theraband resisted diagonally Symmetric internal rotation	Figures 14, A & B	
Chest press	Figure 15E	Pectoralis major and minor, anterior deltoid
Bench press	Figure 16E	Pectoralis major and minor, anterior deltoid
Incline dumbbell press	Figure 16F	Anterior deltoids, pectoralis major and minor, serratus anterior
Chest flyes & chest flyes while on a Swiss gym ball	Figures 16D & 20D	Pectoralis major and minor
Supine reciprocal arm raises while on a Swiss gym ball	Figure 20E	Anterior deltoids, pectoralis major and minor, serratus anterior
Initial and final positions: Upright rowing	Figures 18, A & B	Deltoid, pectoralis major and minor
Reciprocal arm and anterior deltoid arm raises	Figures 17, A & B, 19B	Anterior deltoids
Lateral deltoid raises	Figure 19A	Middle deltoids
Prone reciprocal arm raise	Figure 20A	Posterior deltoid
Supraspinatus raises in standing position	Figure 17D	Supraspinatus
Theraband resisted diagonal internal rotations	Figures 13G & 14D	Pectoralis major, subscrapularis
Theraband resisted diagonal external rotations	Figures 13F & 14C	Infraspinatus

* Note: Co-contraction of direct cervical and thoracolumbar stabilizers must accompany these exercise routines.

TABLE 5.   Interscapular Muscle Strengthening Exercises Useful in Cervicothoracic Stabilization Training*

Interscapular Muscle Strengthening Exercises	Figures	Primary Muscle Groups
Seated rowing	Figure 15A	Latissimus dorsi, rhomboids, middle trapezius, posterior deltoid
Theraband resisted rowing while standing and rowing from a low pulley while standing	Figures 13A & 15B	Trapezius
Theraband resisted pulldown and closed hand pulldown	Figures 13B & 15C	Serratus anterior, latissimus dorsi
Theraband resisted pulldown	Figure 13C	Serratus anterior, latissimus dorsi
Open hand pulldown	Figure 15D	Latissimus dorsi, rhomboids, middle trapezius, posterior deltoid
Incline prone flyes: final position	Figures 16, A & B	Rhomboids, middle trapezius, thoracic lumbar paraspinals
Prone flyes, bilateral arm raises while on a Swiss gym ball and prone flyes while on a Swiss gym ball	Figures, 16C, 20, A & B	Rhomboids, middle trapezius, thoracic lumbar paraspinals
Prone reciprocal arm raise while on a Swiss gym ball	Figure 20A	Rhomboids, middle trapezius, thoracic lumbar paraspinals
Reverse flyes while standing in a flexed hip-hinge position	Figure 17C	Rhomboids, middle trapezius, thoracic lumbar paraspinals

* Note: Co-contraction of direct cervical and thoracolumbar stabilizers must accompany these exercise routines.

TABLE 6. Upper Extremity Muscle Strengthening Exercises Useful for Cervicothoracic Stabilization Training*

Upper Extremity Muscle Strengthening Exercises	Primary Muscle Groups
Biceps pulldown	Biceps brachii
Standing biceps curl	Biceps
Standing triceps press	Triceps brachii

* Note: Co-contraction of direct cervical and thoracolumbar stabilizers must accompany these exercise routines.

REFERENCES

1. Basmajian JV (ed): Therapeutic Exercise. Baltimore, Williams & Wilkins, 1984.
2. Bland JH: Disorders of the Cervical Spine. Philadelphia, W.B. Saunders, 1987.
3. Caplan D: Back Trouble: A New Approach to Prevention and Recovery. Gainesville, FL, Triad Publishing Company, 1987.
4. Foreman SM, Croft AC: Whiplash Injuries: The Cervical Spine Acceleration Deceleration Syndrome. Baltimore, Williams & Wilkins, 1988.
5. Gorman D: The Body Moveable, Vol. I: The Trunk and Head.
6. Gracovetsky S: The Spinal Engine. New York, Springer-Verlag, 1988.
7. Gracovetsky S, Farfan H: The optimum spine. Spine 10:543–573, 1986.
8. Gustavsen R: Training Therapy: Prophylaxis and Rehabilitation. New York, Thieme, 1985.
9. Knott M, Voss D: Proprioceptive Neuromuscular Facilitation: Patterns and Techniques. New York, McGraw-Hill, 1956.
10. Saal JS: Nonoperative treatment of lumbar pain syndromes. In White AH, Anderson R (eds): Conservative Care of Lumbar Spine. Baltimore, Williams & Wilkins (in press).
11. Saal JS: Flexibility training. Physical Medicine and Rehabilitation: State of the Art Reviews 1:537–554, 1987. Philadelphia, Hanley & Belfus, Inc.

STUART M. WEINSTEIN, MD
STANLEY A. HERRING, MD
JOHN L. SHELTON, PhD

THE INJURED WORKER: ASSESSMENT AND TREATMENT

From Puget Sound Sports
  Physicians, Inc.
Seattle, Washington

Reprint requests to:
Stuart Weinstein, MD
Puget Sound Sports
  Physicians, Inc.
4500 Sand Point Way Northeast
Suite 222
Seattle, WA 98105-3914

There are very few non–life-threatening illnesses that generate as much emotion in the health care provider as does back pain in the injured worker. Frustration, anxiety, and anger can and do frequently influence the effectiveness of an evaluation and treatment program. The training of physicians emphasizes objective assessment of illness and injury; emotional feelings should not interfere in patient care. This dictum usually bears truth. However, this distinct patient population, the injured worker with back pain, demands a re-analysis of how one approaches a disease process. Not until the physician, or other provider of care for industrial back pain, appreciates how and why emotional barriers develop when a potential workers' compensation patient enters his or her clinic will effective assessment and management of this disability occur.

Recent reviews have been published describing and documenting the financial burden to society in managing a nonemployed injured worker.[24,44,45,67,69,74,77] As health care providers, we are aware of these sobering statistics, but this does not always influence our clinical judgment. Rather, it is usually the uncertainty of diagnosis, the rate and extent of recovery, and especially patient-provider trust[5] that are foremost in our thoughts. We are concerned about the "hysteric" patient because it is difficult for some practitioners to develop an effective patient relationship with such emotional patients. But it is the malingerer, albeit rare, that is frequently of most concern, as nobody is prepared to be fooled. An early post-World War II paper poignantly describes the development of hysteria, disability, and malingering in the injured worker or soldier, perpetuated by circumstances beyond the physician's immediate control, i.e., the compensation system.[47] Kennedy makes a thought-provoking observation that minimal observable injuries often lead to the most ingrained disability. Whether or not an injury must be observed to be believed is controversial; nevertheless, the lack of objective evidence becomes the crux of many a contested compensation case. Increasingly today, physicians' practice patterns, especially regarding the injured worker, are scrutinized, tending to agitate an already unsettled situation. The demand, therefore, is for early and accurate diagnosis to be made, such that appropriate intervention can be instituted quickly. In this regard, many of the rules and principles of investigating and managing back pain in the patient with a non–work-related injury do not apply to the injured worker. Extensive diagnostic testing performed early may be helpful in allaying patient fears and promoting early return to work, or in predicting those patients at high risk for delayed recovery and for considering early comprehensive pain management treatment.

This chapter is divided into several sections. The first section discusses the scope of the problem and reviews several cost-impact studies as demonstrable examples. Next is an epidemiologic and behavior profile of the stereotypical injured worker. The third section addresses the assessment and diagnostic evaluation of the injured worker, including medical, radiological, and psychosocial evaluations, with emphasis on the risk factors for developing disability and chronic pain syndrome. Lastly, management of the worker with back pain is discussed, including goals, pre-employment screening, nonsurgical and surgical treatment, comprehensive pain management, and the role of managed health care.

SCOPE/COST-IMPACT STUDIES

Industrial back pain is a worldwide epidemic.[2,71] In the U.S., it is estimated that 2% of the national work force per year will sustain a work-related back injury leading to compensation.[11,51] The staggering cost to society of these back injuries reflects not only direct costs such as medical care expenses and time-loss/lost wage payments, but indirect costs referable to production loss and subsequent increased consumer costs, expense of replacing or retraining employees (including the injured worker), and the seemingly endless process of litigation. This is compounded by the observation that return-to-work rates decrease to 50% if the injured worker is off for 6 months, 25% if off for 1 year, and nearly 0% if the worker has not returned to employment by 2 years.[57]

An early study of the occurrence of industrial low back pain was reported by Rowe.[63] This retrospective evaluation of 10 years of medical records from Eastman Kodak Company revealed that 30% of sedentary workers and 47% of heavy handlers had been evaluated for low back pain, with lost time per worker second only to upper respiratory infections. Klein et al. reported labor statistics for 1979 from 26 states.[50] Nineteen percent of all claims filed for worker compensation related to back pain, 86% of these for back sprain/strain, for a total of 285,000 cases. The average medical cost per case was $470, but the average compensation amounted to $3,063. The average direct cost for back injured workers in these 26 states amounted to greater than one billion dollars.

Insurance data reported by Snook in 1985 indicated that for eight states the average compensation claim cost $5,739—one third for medical care and two thirds for time-loss payments. Another study by Holbrook that extrapolated the costs from several national health surveys for the year 1977, estimated that sixteen billion dollars of direct cost would be spent on industrial back pain in 1984.[67]

A recent comprehensive, retrospective study of workers at the Boeing Company in Washington state again demonstrated that back injury claims accounted for approximately 20% of all claims.[69] The number of patients with multiple claims was greater in the back-injured workers. The mean cost of these claims was $2,054, about three times higher than non-back injuries. The total cost amounted to $1.85 million or 41% of the cost of all claims combined. Only 1% of these back injury claims were greater than $10,000, but they amounted to 27% of the cost for all claims, i.e., a very small percentage of the claims was responsible for the majority of expenses. The 10% most expensive claims represented 79% of the total expenses for back injury and 32% of all expenses for all types of injuries.

Other cost-impact studies can be found.[72,80] Clearly the trend is to higher absolute numbers of industrial back injury claims, greater direct and potentially indirect expenses per claim, and a disproportionately large amount of dollars spent on relatively few claims. This latter fact may reflect the prolonged nature of litigation as well as permanent partial disability awards.

Workers' Compensation

The workers' compensation laws were legislated in most of the U.S. in 1949.[37] They were designed as a "no-fault" system, allowing the worker injured in the course of employment and by accidental means to be compensated for permanent partial injury and lost wages. In the course of 40 years, legal embroilments have flourished. Questions arise as to: What is the reasonable risk that an employee assumes in accepting a job if he or she is "injured" without a distinct precipitant? How should preexistent conditions influence compensation following a work injury? And is there a causal relationship between specific work activities and work injuries? More and more physicians are requested to determine disability ratings—sentencing if you will—as patients and their attorneys wait anxiously for the ruling. Most physicians abhor this task, as there is little scientific basis for such decision-making. In the long run the consumers bear the brunt of the cost.

In the U.S. many studies suggest that increased compensation may actually increase the rate of injury.[77] Duration of time loss has also been shown to be prolonged in cases of compensation; injured workers were unable to return to work for 4.9 months versus 3.6 months for non–work-injured workers.[65] The recovery period post-surgery was also greater in the work-injured compensated patient.[65,77] Carron performed interesting comparisons of the compensation system in the United States and New Zealand.[16] The New Zealand compensation/disability/rehabilitation system truly encompasses a no-fault payment plan, as workers are paid a percentage of lost wages whether injured at work or not. This is considered an "entitlement system" as opposed to the "adversarial system" born from the U.S. workers' compensation laws. In an entitlement system there exists little need for litigation, as the onus of proof that an accident truly did occur is not placed on the worker's shoulders. Physicians do not need to address the issue of causality. Early rehabilitation for chronic injuries (greater than 13 weeks) is based on a return-to-work plan that, if not accepted, can lead to significant financial penalty. Carron's data further demonstrate that the percentage of patients receiving compensation for back pain, even prior to treatment, is lower in the New Zealand system. In contrast, open-ended compensation, as in the U.S. system, prolongs disability. Disability for some injured workers becomes the "path of least resistance."

Frequently the chronic low back-injured worker has few objective physical signs to corroborate his or her pain complaints. Persistent symptoms without supportive physical findings, and even nonorganic signs,[76] often result in a label of low back "loser,"[70] malingerer, or compensation neurotic.[47] Secondary gain has long been implicated as a cause of delayed or prolonged recovery from industrial injury.[21,28] Personal experience of the authors suggests that true malingering is rare. Preventing compensation claims, therefore, demands an understanding of the stereotypical injured worker who has the potential for long-term disability.

EPIDEMIOLOGIC AND BEHAVIORAL PROFILE OF THE INJURED WORKER

Many studies in the literature, mostly retrospective reviews, address epidemiologic factors associated with low back pain.[2,6,8,9,13,33,34,45,46,71] A stereotypical profile of the injured worker can be gleaned from these data. Data such as these have an historical interest, can assist in predicting patients at risk for developing prolonged disability, and ultimately can assist in designing prevention and ergonomic screening programs. Kelsey et al. have reported that for the years 1969–70 back pain was the most common chronic condition limiting activity and negatively impacting work capacity in people less than 45 years of age.[45] Most reports of work injury-related factors suggest an age range of 25–40 years,[2,9,50] which does not significantly differ from incidence of back pain in the general population. Bigos et al., in their study of Boeing workers, found that risk of back injury increased below age 25, but the highest compensation claims occurred in workers between 30 and 40 years of age.[9] Most studies suggest that males are injured more frequently than females, but this may reflect the relative number of each in heavy occupations, since in health profession occupations, where females predominate, the reverse can be seen.[13]

The most common workplace activity associated with back injury appears to be handling materials, especially lifting.[2,6,8,13,34,45,50,65,71,80] Lifting greater than 25 pounds, especially if associated with bending or twisting,[45] or self-determined "improper" technique,[8] or lifting boxes,[50] seems to predict higher risk for injury. The Boeing study found that falls placed patients at high risk for higher cost claims (greater than $10,000). Studies regarding vibration have implicated this as an occupational hazard.[33,35] An exogenous frequency of 5 Hz appeared to cause the greatest enhancement of vibrational effect through the spinal-musculoskeletal system. Most industrial and constructional vehicles generate frequencies ranging from 3.5 to 8.9 Hz. Vibrational trauma has been associated with an increased incidence of herniated lumbar discs.

Several occupations have been noted to have the highest rate of compensable back injury, including truck driving (especially loading and unloading), material handling, and the nursing profession.[34,45,50,80] Other work-associated factors are predictive of back injury with potential for delayed recovery. These include low job satisfaction;[6] monotonous, boring or repetitive work;[8,71] a relatively new employee;[9] and a recent poor job rating by a supervisor.[9] It is worthwhile to note that many chronic pain patients are injured workers with delayed recovery and other compensation issues. Our clinical experience reveals several common identifiable traits seen in this patient population that can aid in diagnosis. The duration of pain is often months to years. By definition, we use a period of 3 months to define a chronic problem. Usually, the intensity of pain in these patients is subjectively as high if not higher than upon initial presentation. Previous treatment has often been unsuccessful or has exaggerated symptoms. It is often difficult to determine the exact cause of the ongoing problem. Disability tends to be in excess of that warranted by objective physical findings. There is frequently a psychological trait involved, with elements of anger, depression, high stress, or a general high state of emotional arousal. The likelihood of using or abusing medication is high. Chronic pain patients have goals that tend to be unrealistic. Finally, many physicians evaluating or treating chronic pain patients also have unrealistic goals, and herein may lie a major treatment failure contributing to the cycle of physician apathy and distrust.

MEDICAL ASSESSMENT

Historically, the exact etiology of low back pain has been elusive and specificity of diagnosis reportedly unobtainable in up to 85% of patients with idiopathic low back pain.[24,80] Often, in the worker with a back injury, generic diagnoses are derived. Low back sprain or strain is the most common initial diagnosis of "mechanical" low back pain,[8,23,50,51] and although time and/or testing may elucidate distinct structural abnormalities, the clinical significance of these has been questioned.[24,38,81,84]

Frequently the primary care physician is not trained in the complexities of low back pain. This can lead to the early, unchecked ordering of tests in hopes of demonstrating, and sometimes documenting for compensation reasons, disease. Unfortunately, radiographic abnormalities often poorly correlate with patients' signs and symptoms. At times, early diagnostic intervention is very helpful; however, the physician must be able to interpret imaging studies in the context of the degenerative spinal cascade that occurs over time.[48] Superimpose on this poor communication, and delayed recovery can be predicted to be a likely consequence leading to higher compensation claims.

Assuming referral patterns of injured workers remain unchanged in most communities, the nonspecialist primary care physician must be able to assess the acutely injured worker or worker with chronic pain with specific predefined goals rather than search for specific diagnoses. Low back algorithms have been proposed.[23,83] These follow the basic tenets of medical school curricula, emphasizing the history and physical examination. This requires conscientious questioning, which can be supplemented by preprepared "spinal questionnaires," including detailed review of systems. The goals of such an evaluation include (1) ruling out an extraspinal or systemic source of pain; (2) evaluation for neurogenic impairment that might require emergent surgical consideration; and (3) deciding whether treatment would be altered no matter what the structural pain generator may be. Subsequent diagnostic testing is dependent upon meeting certain criteria.

As stated earlier, emotional reactions are common when evaluating an injured worker. Despite concerns of dramatization or even malingering, the physician must objectively rule out medical conditions or surgical emergencies while being cognizant of potential chronic pain and disability characteristics. Acutely injured workers with back pain are unlikely to have at initial presentation tumor, infection, or inflammatory spondyloarthropathy. Several key points of medical history should, however, be red flags to the physician. One potential surgical emergency is the cauda equina syndrome, which presents with bilateral, often asymmetrical, lower extremity paresis, sensory loss in a saddle distribution, and bowel or bladder dysfunction. Beyond this, there are relatively few conditions, other than severe trauma, that require immediate surgical attention. Even severe radiculopathy with motor deficits (i.e., foot drop) can frequently improve with thoughtful, nonsurgical treatment. It has been our experience that nonprogressive weakness can be monitored for approximately 1 month before further diagnostic testing and other intervention may be necessary, assuming absence of other underlying medical conditions or significant pain. Uncommonly does an acutely injured worker present with back pain signifying systemic or nonspinal disease. However, a history of fevers, unintentional weight loss, prior cancer, or age greater than 50 should all indicate the need for further evaluation for cancer (metastatic or primary) or infection (discitis or osteomyelitis).

Radiography. The use of diagnostic x-rays is controversial. This is well reviewed by Hall.[38] It is commonly suggested that standard, plain, lumbosacral x-rays are not indicated in an acute setting unless fracture, infection, tumor, or sacroiliitis are being considered.[24] Further, limiting studies to AP and lateral views has been shown to significantly reduce radiation exposure and not to decrease the sensitivity of the examination. Oblique x-rays may be ordered in selected cases after reviewing the AP and lateral. The correlation between spine x-ray abnormalities and clinical symptoms has been questioned, with only spondylolisthesis (moderate to severe), multisegmental severe disc-space narrowing, ankylosing spondylitis, severe scoliosis, osteoporosis, congenital kyphosis, or Scheuermann's disease very likely to be associated with pain.[81] CT scans have also been shown to have a low specificity, i.e., a high degree of false positives. Wiesel has demonstrated that 35% of asymptomatic individuals had radiologist-reported abnormalities on CT scan, 19% of patients under 40 diagnosed with herniated nucleus pulposus and greater than 50% of people over 40 having diagnoses of degenerative facet disease or spinal stenosis.[84] Acute, recurrent back pain may be an indication for x-ray imaging, as would a history of immunosuppression, treatment with corticosteroids, or drug or alcohol abuse. Concern regarding loss of patient trust when x-rays are not ordered immediately may be unwarranted.[26]

Blood Tests. Routine ordering of blood tests has also been discouraged in the acute setting. The erythrocyte sedimentation rate has been demonstrated to help differentiate between patients with and without neoplasms. Thus, the ESR has been suggested as the one useful blood test to be ordered early. Although highly sensitive, the ESR is fairly nonspecific, so that an abnormality may indicate the need for additional spinal imaging studies and/or further medical workup.

Other Diagnostic Concerns. The evaluation of an injured worker with chronic back pain raises additional concerns. Frequently it is a consultant who may be asked to render an opinion. Objectivity is important and initial "labeling" should be avoided. A higher index of suspicion for potentially missed diagnoses is important. In this regard additional diagnostic evaluation may be warranted including imaging studies (MRI, CT/myelogram, bone scan), electromyography/nerve conduction studies, blood work-up (ESR, C-reactive protein, CBC) and selective spinal injections (including nerve root block, epidural steroid injection, and facet joint injection). Commonly missed diagnoses include dynamic lateral nerve entrapment, lateral recess stenosis, far-lateral disc herniation, internal disc disruption, primary radiculitis, inflammatory conditions, and occult facet or lamina injury. Although it has been suggested that the extent of pathoanatomy is poorly correlated with ultimate claim costs,[52] one should be aware of the relatively low level of diagnostic acumen in most primary care physicians. However, this should not automatically indicate the need for surgical consultation.[11,53] Indeed, the value of a surgical consultant in a work-injured, chronic back pain patient is questionable. The benefits of surgical treatment in chronic pain patients have been shown to be low.[1] Further, lacking specific case management, disability is usually perpetuated.

PSYCHOLOGICAL ASSESSMENT AND RISK FACTORS

Functional assessment, regarding disability and not simply nonorganicity, must be included in any evaluation of a chronic pain patient who may be at high risk for delayed recovery. Early psychological assessment can be invaluable in identifying these high-risk patients and can assist the primary care physician or consultant.[35] The task of identifying the high-risk patient, however, is not an easy one. Over the years a number of researchers have struggled with this issue with only marginal results. Recently progress has begun in this important area of investigation. Led by the efforts of Cats-Baril and Frymoyer, important research is now being published that, for the first time, enables one to identify high-risk patients with a high degree of accuracy.[18] What follows are our views on the identification of high-risk patients. Our position with regard to risk indicators is based on available published research and our own research efforts as well as our own clinical observations.

A great deal can be accomplished in identifying the presence or absence of risk factors by carefully observing the patient during the initial intake examination. Physicians should be particularly sensitive to instances of intense and exaggerated pain behavior and descriptions of pain that use nonphysiologic words such as "terrible," "frustrating," and "murderous." Careful attention should be directed at the spouse of the patient, if present, to note overly responsive behavior, speaking for the patient, and prompts on the spouse's part to ensure that the patient tells the most alarming story possible. Injured patients with disabled spouses represent a particularly potent mix regarding their inability to successfully navigate the health care system and promptly return to work. Patients with subacute difficulties, those lasting 6 to 12 weeks, who ask for medications immediately, should also be viewed with suspicion. Similarly, patients with a history of substance abuse frequently lead to protracted medical care with little result. Patients with a protracted history of previous injuries and relative failure to respond to treatments offered should also be viewed with caution. The best measure of future behavior is past events.

Careful observation should also be made regarding patient's emotional status. Anger, especially when directed at the insurance system or the previous employer for perceived fault in causing the injury, has high predictive power regarding prolonged recovery.[32] Self-reported elevated pain levels should be viewed with suspicion. Although it is hard to specify an exact numerical cutoff point, our research, using a visual analogue measure, suggests that patients' reports of pains exceeding 7 on a 10-point scale often suggest prolonged recovery. Cats-Baril and Frymoyer report similar results.[18]

Occupational Issues

Frymoyer and Cats-Baril have provided evidence to show that occupational issues are the single most important variable when detecting patients at high risk for slow movement through the health care system.[32] Interestingly, their initial research found medical issues to be only the third most important, behind occupational and psychological issues, when detecting high-risk patients.

The patient's occupational status often plays a rather profound role in the determination of whether or not the rehabilitation goals are reached. A number of variables within the general rubric of occupation have been shown to influence recovery. Perhaps the most important of these is the amount of time off work. Similar to statistics presented earlier in this chapter, Beals' data are representative of the typical findings.[4] Patients off work for more than 6 months have only a 50% chance of ever returning to work in their lifetime. Those injured and off work for 1 year have only a 10% chance of ever returning to work, and those off work for 2 years or more have virtually no chance of ever returning without highly coordinated and well integrated efforts, such as those provided in pain clinics. Physicians attempting to provide solo treatment for injured workers off work for more than 1 year are virtually doomed to failure.

Closely related to time off work is the issue of whether or not the patient has a job waiting. Employers having "light duty" or "modified jobs" available for injured workers can sometimes play a critical role in eventual rehabilitation and return to work. Patients who have a job waiting often have incentive to put forth vigorous efforts in rehabilitation, whereas those with little or no incentive often fail to progress satisfactorily.

Other occupational issues are important as well. As previously mentioned, the risk of low-back disability is directly related to a number of high-risk occupations, such as truck driving and nursing.[44] This appears to particularly be the case if there is a mismatch between the demands of the job and the patient's physical capacity. Of considerable interest is the fact that Bigos has shown that the patient's perception of this mismatch is enough to warrant the possibility of a high-risk status.[7] Further, dissatisfaction with one's job has potential high risk for injury and time loss.

Litigation. It is generally believed that the involvement of an attorney with the injured patient frequently adds to the likelihood of the development of long-term disability and protracted treatment.[77] According to Wiesel et al., chronic pain is frequently found among litigants.[82] Their observations suggest that litigants exaggerate the severity of pain and perpetuate disability in order to maximize the financial gains that are eventually awarded. However, research findings in this regard are by no means unanimous. Mendelson has pointed out some of the difficulties with studies in this important area.[59]

A closely related area is that of compensation or litigation for an injury. Although the results of investigations in this area are mixed,[59] it is generally believed that compensation or litigation for injuries is a negative sign regarding the rapidity by which injured workers move through the health care system.[10,29,40,70]

Other Factors. Educational background and in particular English proficiency are variables that can predict the inability to profit from rehabilitation efforts designed to enable the patient to return to work.[25] Other factors such as sex and age of the patients have no clear-cut predictive basis regarding return to work.

These high-risk variables are summarized in Table 1.

MANAGEMENT OF LOW BACK PAIN

Conservative Approach. Conservative treatment has in general remained the accepted norm for treating acute low back pain. In some instances, such as acute cauda equina syndrome, the "conservative" treatment may indeed be

TABLE 1. Summary of Most Predictive Risk Factors for Delayed Recovery

1. Physician's conviction of extreme high-risk status.
2. Poor English proficiency.
3. Time off work.
4. Job satisfaction.
5. Patient's perception of heavy work.
6. Physician's perception of heavy work.
7. Anger at system—excessive fault finding.
8. Substance abuse.
9. Previous injuries.
10. Spouse disabled.

surgical decompression. Usually, however, conservative equates with nonsurgical. A review of the use of various therapeutic agents in treating acute back pain, including modalities, traction, manipulation, and electrical stimulation, demonstrated how little scientific data is available to clearly state that any of these facilitate recovery.[22] This is supported by the well-accepted fact that 90% or greater of the people with acute low back pain will be pain free by 3 months, and only 1 to 2% of back injured workers ultimately require surgical intervention. Nevertheless, the rehabilitation of an acutely injured worker with back pain should follow general principles of musculoskeletal medicine, including rest,[27] anti-inflammatory measures, and progressive exercise through a physical therapy program. Flexibility and strengthening exercises of some form[58,62] have fairly universal acceptance as a part of recovery from a back injury.

Improved fitness has been recognized to protect certain workers with high physical demand from back injury.[14] Specific muscular strengthening through techniques of truncal stabilization has been recognized as an effective means of protecting the spinal segments from shear or rotational stress.[64] Such strengthening may play a role in protecting the injured spine from reoccurrence when returning workers to repetitive bending, lifting, and twisting jobs. Epidural steroid injection may also have a role in the acutely injured worker with suspected disc protrusion or herniation, with or without the presence of radicular symptoms.[43] There is some evidence, however, that epidural steroid injections in back-injured workers with outstanding compensation issues may respond less well than the back-injured patient who has no work-related injuries.[78] This supports our clinical experience, and indeed relatively few selective spinal injections are performed on back-injured workers with chronic pain. Occasionally, however, selective injection can reveal and treat previously undiagnosed disease, such as an atypical presentation of radiculopathy, in patients with chronic back pain.

Surgical Intervention. The results of surgical intervention in this same chronic pain population are frequently poor. Beals has reported that return to work becomes less likely as the number of operations increased, especially after three surgical procedures.[4] Akeson has suggested that there exists only a 30% chance of successful outcome in a chronic pain patient and only 5% following two or more surgeries.[1] Results from spinal fusion are also less likely to be "satisfactory" in patients with outstanding compensation or litigation issues. Turner reported that following lumbosacral fusion, 86% of noncompensation patients had satisfactory results (including return to work) as compared to 48% satisfactory results in compensation patients.[73] Further, spinal fusion tends to occur several years after the time of injury, and frequently several surgeries have already been performed. It is our experience that the patient with a multioperated spine undergoing spinal fusion is even less likely to return to work.

Orthoses.   In certain subsets of injured workers with chronic back pain we have utilized external stabilization via the Boston Overlap Brace. This is usually in instances of chronic nonradiating pain with or without documented instability on lateral flexion-extension x-rays. Presumably, some degree of segmental hypermobility, possibly due to internal disc disruption, may exist, and neutral spine stabilization exercises in physical therapy have failed. These braces may be worn for as long as 3 to 6 months during all waking hours. Initial data appear to suggest that pain reduction and improved function result. Data on long-term return to work are not yet available. Activity and specific stabilization strengthening exercises are encouraged in the brace. Early return to work is promoted.

Ergonomic Intervention.   Another method of managing industrial back pain is through prevention and ergonomic assessment. Occupational risk factors contributing to back injury have been previously outlined. Manual handling, including lifting, pushing, pulling and carrying, accounts for up to 70% of all injuries in some studies.[8,66,68] Modifying job sites with improved work-space design and addition of mechanical aids has been shown to decrease both the incidence and cost of back injuries.[66] Such alteration can also accommodate for excessive twisting and bending, prolonged sitting, and vibration. Preemployment screening evaluations have been suggested, including history and physical examination, radiography, and strength testing.[19,57,66,68] Historical information can be helpful if a previous history of back pain is uncovered, as risk of recurrence is high; otherwise, little benefit is derived from the preemployment history and physical. Use of screening radiographs has been controversial.[36,57] Preemployment strength testing is discussed in detail in the article on p. 271.

Back Schools.   Back schools have been used as a preventative aid. Most are modeled after the Swedish back school, including lectures, exercising, ergonomic counseling, and actual demonstrations.[87] The effectiveness of back schools alone is questionable.[12] Logic would suggest that education and training in such areas as proper lifting and bending would decrease the incidence of back injury; however, carry-over, compliance and application of these skills are problematic. There are few well-controlled studies available. Further, it is frequently the inexperienced or new employee that may require more selective training.[49,66,68] In a study of patients with very chronic pain, not solely injured workers, it was demonstrated that the equivalent of a Swedish back school could reduce pain and functional disability, whereas exercise alone was ineffective.[49] Indeed, rehabilitation of the acutely injured lumbosacral spine should extend beyond relief of symptoms. Addressing flexibility, strengthening, body mechanics, and education following acute care has a biomechanical and epidemiological rationale. Perhaps the 70 to 90% recurrence rate of back pain episodes could be decreased.[20,41,42]

Chronic Back Pain Worker

Most injured workers will return to work within 2 to 3 months following an injury. As reported, it is the chronic back pain worker who imparts the greatest socioeconomic drain on the system. In the acute setting, pain alleviation is the prime focus of both the patient and physician. Unfortunately, in patients with chronic back pain, many primary care physicians are also driven to provide symptomatic pain relief. This is usually unsuccessful and may contribute to further psychological impairment and disability through the prescription of centrally acting medication such as narcotic analgesics and muscle antispasmodics.

The management of chronic back pain in the disabled worker is multifactorial.[3,31,74] Such comprehensive treatment implies that the classic medical model of disease does not apply; rather, treatment is focused on a biopsychosocial process. Nociception, defined as the peripheral, afferent neuronal response to a potentially damaging stimulus, is usually absent. This chronic pain syndrome has at its core a combination of subjective complaints of pain ("centrally" mediated), psychological distress and suffering (negative affective response), and magnified illness or pain behavior, that is out of proportion to underlying pathophysiology.[31,60,75] This is supported by the observation that the pathologic disorder has not been shown to be predictive of outcome from such a multidisciplinary pain management program,[15] and most comprehensive programs emphasize behavioral modification principles as a component of rehabilitation.[29-31] Pain behavior is an externally measurable response. It includes observations of postural alteration, facial expression, verbalization, medication use, compensation, etc. These behaviors can be both reinforced or extinguished through conditioning.

In the past 10 to 15 years, hundreds of "pain clinics" have arisen in the U.S. Many of these centers have as their purpose simply to treat pain through various techniques such as acupuncture, electrostimulation, manipulation, injection, biofeedback, and the sort. However, concomitant with chronic pain is deconditioning, depression, job skill reduction, impaired coping skills, and inability to work. Consequently, many work-hardening programs have been developed. Although these programs can affect deconditioning, frequently important psychosocial issues are not addressed. True multidisciplinary pain clinics, therefore, strive for several distinct goals: (1) improved function for usual activities of daily living; (2) early return to work; (3) discontinued utilization of the health care system; and (4) control of pain, both as a consequence of the first three and through other more direct means. How well individual clinics may meet these goals varies with the nature of the selected patients as well as the skills of the individual team members. Outcome measures cannot simply be based on reduction in reports of pain. Functional outcomes such as return to work may be more quantitative, although they too are subject to multiple exogenous factors, including the presence of compensation.[77]

The team approach to treating chronic pain in the injured worker exists on two levels. One incorporates the patient's environment, especially family, into his or her treatment program. Family members can not only positively reinforce pain behavior, but also can be instrumental in altering behavior. The second level of interdisciplinary involvement is the members of the team. Usually this includes a physician, physical and occupational therapists, psychologist, vocational counselor, and frequently a social worker or nurse. The intrateam dynamics of a pain clinic will not be described here. However, several key issues are addressed regarding the role of the psychologist in evaluating and treating chronic back-injured patients.

Psychological Management

An initial premise of this chapter was that back-injured patients generate a significant emotional response in the evaluating physician. Uneasiness about expected recovery in this potentially litigious/compensable population occurs. The experienced physician may have a "gut reaction" of high-risk status for delayed recovery. In such cases early referral for pscyhobehavioral evaluation is appropriate.

The typical 30-minute initial examination or 15-minute recheck does not permit the in-depth questioning and observation that is needed to provide solid objective content to support the physician's high-risk hypothesis.

The clinical psychologist or psychiatrist can provide further vital functions as well. An overworked treating physician, who must track thousands of details for hundreds of patients, can overlook the difficulties involved in communicating complex issues when talking to a patient with poor English proficiency as a result of a meager educational background. Add to this the fact that discussions involving pain can be emotionally arousing makes it very likely that miscommunication will occur. In many instances, this miscommunication can cause noncompliance, depression, and anger on the part of the patient. Frustration and burnout on the physician's part can occur because of numerous follow-up phone calls, all aimed at issues perceived by the physician to have been discussed in full during the last recheck meeting. Having a rehabilitation psychologist as part of the team allows misunderstandings to be cleared up before they grow into heated issues between doctor and patient. On some occasions, the team psychologist is actually in attendance during recheck meetings. On other occasions, he is able to talk directly with the attending physician in order to clarify issues that are then addressed during the next treatment session.

The psychologist, in addition to assisting in the identification of high-risk patients and smoothing out communication between doctor and patient, can alert the attending physician to a wide number of factors that have the potential to interrupt a well-designed rehabilitation plan. Medication and alcohol abuse, family difficulties, poor coping skill, secondary gains, and issues related to ongoing litigation can all be addressed and communicated to the attending physician in order to make his or her influence more sizable.

Psychological evaluation can be pursued independent of a formal pain clinic, especially in the acutely injured worker. The psychologist-physician team can be enhanced by having the psychologist physically present on the premises. Ease of patient referral and communication of critical medical and "emotional" data are pluses. The traditional model of time-consuming and inefficient letter-writing and infrequent, frustrating telephone calls regarding these complex patients can be bypassed. This office model, however, has limitations, namely compensable chronic pain syndrome requires an even higher intensity of intervention, and the referring physician must be experienced in chronic pain management. Difficult-to-manage patients should on occasion be considered for pain clinic referral. Patients with obvious medication, alcohol, or street drug abuse top the list. Those with excessive pain behavior or patients with a history of noncompliance are also candidates for comprehensive management.

Pain Clinics

Pain clinic referral is not a treatment of last resort.[3] Early intervention can potentially avoid long delays in recovery, avoid multiple inappropriate surgeries, and despite the relative expense of these programs, actually save money. Patients who have a majority of high-risk factors (see Table 1) should be considered for immediate or early referral. Of all the risk factors listed in various studies, our clinical experience suggests that those in Table 1 are the most predictive of delayed recovery, and are listed in order of predicting "failure" patients.

Given the relative high cost of multidisciplinary pain clinics, especially inpatient programs with durations of 3 to 6 weeks, questions have been raised as to cost effectiveness. Clearly this hinges on outcome results. Criteria for positive outcome include return to work, elimination of compensation or time loss, reduced use of the health care system, increased daily activities, reduction in pain medication usage, and subjective reduction in pain. Few studies, however, have adequate control groups, i.e., treated versus nontreated. Several studies available in the literature were reviewed.[3,15,17,55,56] A review by Aronoff suggests that a "success rate" of greater than 50% return to work is an excellent result. Success frequently depends upon patients' active participation, follow-through, and motivation, although socioeconomic factors such as age, pre-injury skills, and job availability may also play a role. In a study comparing "successful" versus "failure" patients, those who did not actively change their lifestyle and adopt a "self-help" attitude did poorly.[61] Frequently, contracts between patient and program facilitate recovery. Catchlove, in a retrospective evaluation, found that if a directive to return to work within 1 to 2 months following completion of a multidisciplinary program was given in the preliminary stages, a 60% return-to-work rate was found as compared to 25% in the group who did not receive such a directive.[17] Follow-up after approximately 10 months demonstrated that 90% of the "treated" group were still working, received less compensation, and required less medical treatment. The psychological support system of this program was critical in diffusing the anger that commonly occurred as increasingly independent action was required of the patients.

Both inpatient and outpatient pain management programs exist. Inpatient programs tend to be reserved for the more chronic, disability-ingrained patients. This may explain the results of a study by Cairns that demonstrated 90% success in outpatient groups, as indicated by decreased pain complaints and increased activity level 1 year following completion of the program, compared to 50% in the inpatient group.[15] Interestingly, 28% of the patients in the success group still sought further treatment, implying again that pain reduction is not a complete definition of recovery nor a primary goal of chronic pain management programs. Also presented was a multifactorial analysis to determine the likelihood of return to work in inpatient versus outpatient programs. The benefit of such an equation is to avoid potentially unsuccessful treatment programs initially, as each "failure" can lead to further disability and wasted health care dollars.

Functional Restoration. Mayer et al. describe a variation of the classic pain clinic labeled as a functional restoration program.[55,56] This combined features of the traditional pain management program, including psychological support (individual and group counseling, family counseling, stress management, and behavioral modification training), with a physical conditioning program, including strength and endurance training. Objective measures were a major component of this program, including quantitative range of motion, isometric and isokinetic trunk strength evaluation, static and dynamic lifting parameters, and aerobic capacity. All patients were considered medically stable prior to initiation and were encouraged to "work through pain." The nontreated group was denied admission due to various insurance policies. Results after 1 year revealed an 85% return-to-work or retraining rate in the treatment group as compared to 39% in the nontreatment group. At 2 years follow-up, the comparison was 87% to 39%. Additionally, rates of recurrence, further surgeries, and further use of health care practitioners all decreased in the treatment group.

Although comparison data for functional parameters were not available in the nontreatment group, this was considered to be an essential factor in providing feedback and reinforcement to the treatment group.

Managed Health Care.   One of the more recent philosophies in the treatment of back-injured workers is the concept of managed health care for industry. Modification of this concept was utilized in a previous programmed study.[54] Two industrial populations were followed subsequent to sustaining low back injuries. The "active" group received regular evaluations by a neutral physician in addition to the primary care physician, whereas the "passive" group had only one initial evaluation and was seen only if return to work predictions, at initial evaluation, were not realized. Communication and interaction between physicians were critical in the active system, especially if disagreement regarding treatment developed. Treatment followed specific protocols. Both groups demonstrated significant reduction in absolute numbers of patients injured, lost time from work, and compensation costs, although results from the active group were much more impressive. It was concluded that regular, intensive follow-up after work injury was beneficial to both employees and employers.

A Canadian prospective study on the effects of early intervention after work-related back injury also demonstrated significant time and cost savings.[39]

Both of these studies illustrate the value of managing the physician and/or physical therapy aspects of the treatment of the injured worker's back. Even greater decrease of time loss and compensation may be possible if the case management extends between health care providers and industry. The employer must be informed as to the extent of the back injury to the worker, the expected time off work, and necessity of some temporary or permanent restrictions when return to work occurs. This information is useless, however, if the employer has no internal mechanism for management of injured workers. Many companies have no light-duty or parttime return-to-work positions, and there is no incentive for supervisors to reinstate an injured worker. Also cumbersome insurance regulations often impede appropriate medical assessment and treatment, further decreasing the chance for successful early resumption of employment and increasing physician and patient anger and frustration.

Some companies have realized the benefits of coordinating management of the injured worker with the health care team. Prevention seminars and on-site safety assessments are helpful to avoid injury. Determination of the physical capacity requirements of specific jobs and the creation of temporary, less physically taxing positions, make medical treatment easier and more effective.[12] Careful tracking of employees' participation in therapy and progressive return to work programs is also essential. These issues demand a close working relationship between medicine and industry. Several preliminary meetings between a company and physicians providing care must occur and usually a coordinator is needed to track injured employees. The patient must be made to feel as though there is genuine concern for his or her welfare, both medically and vocationally. The physician cannot be perceived as a "company doctor" but rather the patient must feel he or she is receiving quality, expeditious care. The physician must understand low back injury, be willing to take the time to learn details about the particular industry, and be able to identify potential problem patients early. Health care providers and industry together may be able to stem the injured workers' epidemic. Participation of the legal community and labor unions would further serve to slow the runaway problem of work injury and disability.

CONCLUSION

Low back pain in the injured worker is a complex illness. The tangible economic burden of medical and time-loss payments in this patient population is enormous, even before considering the secondary impact of retraining and elevation of consumer costs. Treatment of these patients is difficult, in part due to the emotional reactions and frustration generated in the physician. Implicit in the management of industrial back pain is the necessity of the practitioner to be knowledgeable in spine care, including both acute and chronic pain. However, expertise in management of low back pain is not enought. A working understanding of the industrial health care system is necessary in order to effectively manage low back pain in the injured worker. Recent trends in comprehensive care encourage the active participation of employers with goals of limiting the present extent of compensation and disability.

REFERENCES

1. Akeson WH, Murphy RW: Editorial comments: Low back pain. Clin Orthop 129:2-3, 1979.
2. Andersson GBJ: Epidemiologic aspects on low-back pain in industry. Spine 6:53-60, 1981.
3. Aronoff GM, McAlary PW, Witkower A, et al: Pain treatment programs: Do they return workers to the workplace? SPINE: State Art Rev 2:123-136, 1987.
4. Beals RK, Hickman NY: Industrial injuries of the back and extremities: Comprehensive evaluation—an aid in prognosis and management: A study of one hundred and eighty patients. J Bone Joint Surg 54A:1593-1611, 1972.
5. Behan RC, Hirschfield AH: The accident process: II. Toward more rational treatment of industrial injuries. JAMA 186:84-90, 1963.
6. Bergenudd H, Nilsson B: Back pain in middle age: Occupational work load and psychologic factors: An epidemiologic survey. Spine 13:58-60, 1988.
7. Bigos SJ, Crites Battle M: Acute care to prevent back disability. Clin Orthop 221:121-130, 1987.
8. Bigos SJ, Spengler DM, Martin NA, et al: Back injuries in industry; a retrospective study II. Injury factors. Spine 11:246-251, 1986.
9. Bigos SJ, Spengler DM, Martin NA, et al: Back injuries in industry; a retrospective study III. Employee-related factors. Spine 11:252-256, 1986.
10. Block AR, Kremer E, Gaylor M: Behavioral treatments of chronic pain: Variables affecting treatment efficacy. Pain 8:367-381, 1980.
11. Bond MB: Low back injuries in industry. Indust Med 39:28-32, 1970.
12. Borenstein DG, Wiesel SW: Low Back Pain: Medical Diagnosis and Comprehensive Management. Philadelphia, WB Saunders, 1989, pp 449-514.
13. Brown JR: Factors contributing to the development of low back pain in industrial workers. Am Ind Hyg Assoc J 36:26-31, 1975.
14. Cady LD, Thomas PC, Karwasky RJ: Program for increasing health and fitness of firefighters. J Occup Med 27:110-114, 1985.
15. Carins D, Mooney V, Crane P: Spinal pain rehabilitation: Inpatient and outpatient treatment results and development of predictors for outcome. Spine 9:91-95, 1984.
16. Carron H, DeGood DE, Tait R: A comparison of low back pain patients in the United States and New Zealand: Psychosocial and economic factors affecting severity of disability. Pain 21:77-89, 1985.
17. Catchlove R, Cohen K: Effects of a directive return to work approach in the treatment of workman's compensation patients with chronic pain. Pain 14:181-191, 1982.
18. Cats-Baril W, Frymoyer JW: Identifying patients at risk of becoming disabled due to low back pain: The Vermont Rehabilitation Engineering Center predictive model. Presented at the Eastern Orthopedic Association for Spinal Research, October 1988.
19. Chaffin DB, Herrin GD, Keyserling WM: Preemployment strength testing: An updated position. J Occup Med 20:403-408, 1978.
20. Delin O, Hedenrund B, Horal J: Back symptoms in nursing aides in a geriatric hospital. Scand J Rehabil Med 8:47, 1976.
21. Derebery VJ, Tullis WH: Delayed recovery in the patient with a work compensable injury. J Occup Med 25:829-835, 1983.
22. Deyo RA: Conservative therapy for low back pain. JAMA 250:1057-1062, 1983.

23. Deyo RA: Early diagnostic evaluation of low back pain. J Gen Intern Med 1:328–338, 1986.
24. Deyo RA: The role of the primary care physician in reducing work absenteeism and costs due to back pain. SPINE: State Art Rev 2:17–30, 1987.
25. Deyo RA, Diehl AK: Predicting disability in patients with low back pain. Clin Res 34:814A, 1986.
26. Deyo RA, Diehl AK, Rosenthal M: Reducing x-ray utilization: Can patient expectations be altered? Clin Res 34:814A, 1986.
27. Deyo RA, Diehl AK, Rosenthal M: How many days of bed rest for acute low back pain? a randomized clinical trial. New Engl J Med 315:1064–1070, 1986.
28. Finneson BE: Psychosocial considerations in low back pain: The "cause" and "cure" of industry related low back pain. Orthop Clin North Am 8:23–26, 1977.
29. Fordyce WE: Behavorial Methods for Chronic Back Pain and Illness. St. Louis, CV Mosby, 1976.
30. Fordyce WE, Fowler RS, Lehmann JF, et al: Operant conditioning in the treatment of chronic pain. Arch Phys Med Rehabil 54:399–408, 1973.
31. Fordyce WE, Roberts AH, Sternbach RA: The behavioral management of chronic pain: A response to critics. Pain 22:113–125, 1985.
32. Frymoyer J, Cats-Baril W: Predictors of low back pain disability. Clin Orthop 221:90–97, 1987.
33. Frymoyer J, Pope MH, Clements JH, et al: Risk factors in low-back pain. An epidemiological survey. J Bone Joint Surg 65A:213–218, 1983.
34. Frymoyer JW, Pope MH, Costanza MC, et al: Epidemiologic studies of low-back pain. Spine 5:419–423, 1980.
35. Frymoyer JW, Rosen JC, Clements J, et al: Psychologic factors in low-back-pain disability. Clin Orthop Rel Res 195:178–184, 1985.
36. Gibson ES: The value of preplacement screening radiography of the low back. SPINE: State Art Rev 2:91–107, 1987.
37. Hadler NM: Legal ramifications of the medical definition of back disease. Ann Intern Med 89:992–999, 1978.
38. Hall FM: Back pain and the radiologist. Radiology 137:861–863, 1980.
39. Hall H, Grant P, Hockley B: A controlled prospective study on the effect of early intervention by the Canadian Back Institute on cost and time loss after back injury. Presented at North American Spine Society, Fourth Annual Meeting, Quebec, Canada, June 1989.
40. Hammond W, Brena SF, Unikel LP: Compensation for work related injuries and rehabiliation of patients with chronic pain. South Med J 71:664–666, 1978.
41. Hirsch C, Johnsson R, Lewin J: Low back symptoms in a Swedish female population. Clin Orthop 63:171–176, 1969.
42. Horal J: The clinical appearance of low back disorders in the city of Gothenburg, Sweden. Acta Orthop Scand 118(suppl):8, 1969.
43. Jeffries B: Epidural steroid injections. SPINE: State Art Rev 2:419–426, 1988.
44. Kaplan RM, Deyo RA: Back pain in health care workers. SPINE: State Art Rev 2:61–73, 1987.
45. Kelsey JL, Golden AL: Occupational and workplace factors associated with low back pain. SPINE: State Art Rev 2:61–73, 1987.
46. Kelsey JL, White AA: Epidemiology and impact of low-back pain. Spine 5:133–142, 1980.
47. Kennedy F: The mind of the injured worker. Its effect on disability periods. Compensation Med 1:19–24, 1946.
48. Kirkaldy-Willis WH, Wedge JH, Yong-Hing K, et al: Pathology and pathogenesis of lumbar spondylosis and stenosis. Spine 3:319–328, 1978.
49. Klaber Moffett JA, Chase SM, Portek I, et al: A controlled prospective study to evaluate the effectiveness of a back school in the relief of chronic low back pain. Spine 11:120–122, 1986.
50. Klein BP, Jensen RC, Sanderson LM: Assessment of workers' compensation claims for back strains/sprains. J Occup Med 26:443–448, 1984.
51. Leavitt SS, Johnston TL, Beyer RD: The process of recovery: Patterns in industrial back injury: Part 1. Costs and other quantitative measures of effort. Indust Med 40(8):7–14, 1971.
52. Leavitt SS, Johnston TL, Beyer RD: The process of recovery: Patterns in industrial back injury: Part 2. Predicting outcomes from early case data. Indust Med 40(9):7–15, 1971.
53. Leavitt SS, Johnston TL, Beyer RD: The process of recovery: Patterns in industrial back injury: Part 3. Mapping the health care process. Indust Med 41(1):7–11, 1972.
54. Lonstein MB, Wiesel SW: Standardized approaches to the evaluation and treatment of industrial low back pain. SPINE: State Art Rev 2:147–156, 1987.
55. Mayer TG, Gatchel RJ, Kishino N, et al: Objective assessment of spine function following industrial injury. A prospective study with comparison group and one-year follow-up. Spine 10:482–493, 1985.

56. Mayer TG, Gatchel RJ, Mayer H, et al: A prospective two-year study of functional restoration in industrial low back injury. JAMA 258:1763–1767, 1987.
57. McGill JM: Industrial back problems. A control program. J Occup Med 10:174–178, 1968.
58. McKenzie RA: Prophylaxis in recurrent low back pain. NZ Med J 89:22–23, 1979.
59. Mendelson G: Chronic pain and compensation: A review. J Pain Symp Management 1:135–144, 1986.
60. Nachemson A: Work for all. For those with low back pain as well. Clin Orthop Rel Res 179:77–85, 1983.
61. Painter JR, Seres JL, Newman RI: Assessing benefits of the pain center. Why some patients regress. Pain 8:101–113, 1980.
62. Ponte DJ, Jensen GJ, Kent BE: A preliminary report on the use of the McKenzie protocol versus Williams protocol in the treatment of low back pain. J Orthop Sp Phys Ther 6:130–139, 1984.
63. Rowe ML: Low back pain in industry. A position paper. J Occup Med 11:161–169, 1969.
64. Saal JA: Rehabilitation of sports-related lumbar spine injuries. PHYS MED REHABIL: State Art Rev 1:613–638, 1987.
65. Sander RA, Meyers JE: The relationship of disability to compensation status in railroad workers. Spine 11:141–143, 1986.
66. Snook SH: Approaches to the control of back pain in industry: Job design, job placement and education/training. SPINE: State Art Rev 2:45–59, 1987.
67. Snook SH: The costs of back pain in industry. SPINE: State Art Rev 2:1–5, 1987.
68. Snook SH, Campanelli RA, Hart JW: A study of three preventive approaches to low back injury. J Occup Med 20:478–481, 1978.
69. Spengler DM, Bigos SJ, Martin NA, et al: Back injuries in industry: A retrospective study. I. Overview and cost analysis. Spine 11:241–245, 1986.
70. Sternbach RA, Wolf SR, Murphy RW, et al: Traits of pain patients: The low-back "loser." Psychosomatics 14:226–229, 1973.
71. Svensson HO, Andersson GBJ: Low-back pain in 40- to 47-year-old men: Work history and work environment factors. Spine 8:272–276, 1983.
72. Troup JDG, Martin JW, Lloyd DCEF: Back pain in industry. A prospective survey. Spine 6:61–69, 1981.
73. Turner RS, Leiding WC: Correlation of the MMPI with lumbosacral spine fusion results. Prospective study. Spine 10:932–936, 1985.
74. Waddell G: A new clinical model for the treatment of low-back pain. Spine 12:632–644, 1987.
75. Waddell G, Main CJ, Morris EW, et al: Chronic low-back pain, psychologic distress, and illness behavior. Spine 9:209–213, 1984.
76. Waddell G, McCulloch JA, Kummel E, et al: Nonorganic physical signs in low-back pain. Spine 5:117–125, 1980.
77. Walsh NE, Dumitru L: The influence of compensation on recovery from low back pain. SPINE: State Art Rev 2:109–121, 1987.
78. Warfield CA, Crews DA: Work status and response to epidural steroid injection. J Occup Med 29:315–316, 1987.
79. Westrin D, Hirsch C, Lindegard B: The personality of the back patient. Clin Orthop 87:209–213, 1972.
80. White AA, Gordon SL: Synopsis: Workshop on idiopathic low-back pain. Spine 7:141–149, 1982.
81. White AA, Panjabi MM: Clinical Biomechanics of the Spine. Philadelphia, JB Lippincott, 1978, pp 277–344.
82. Wiesel SW, Feffer HL, Rothman RW: Industrial Low Back Pain. Charlottesville, VA, Michie Company, 1985.
83. Wiesel SW, Feffer HL, Rothman RW: Industrial low-back pain. A prospective evaluation of a standardized diagnostic and treatment protocol. Spine 9:199–203, 1984.
84. Wiesel SW, Tsourmas N, Feffer HL, et al: A study of computer-assisted tomography. I. The incidence of positive CAT scans in an asymptomatic group of patients. Spine 9:549–551, 1984.
85. Wilder DG, Woodworth BB, Frymoyer JW, et al: Vibration and the human spine. Spine 7:243–254, 1982.
86. Wood DJ: Design and evaluation of a back injury prevention program within a geriatric hospital. Spine 12:77–82, 1987.
87. Zachrisson Forssell M: The back school. Spine 6:104, 1981.

JEFFREY A. SAAL, MD

THE FUTURE OF SPINAL MEDICINE

From the San Francisco Spine
  Institute
Daly City, California

Reprint requests to:
Jeffrey A. Saal, MD
Director, Research & Education
San Francisco Spine Institute
1850 Sullivan Ave., #140
Daly City, CA 94015

The controversy surrounding the etiology of lumbar pain continues to rage. Unfortunately, the confusion has led to nihilism and paralysis of creative approaches to understanding this complex situation. Historically, the "low back dilemma" has been unfairly and unwittingly placed upon the shoulders of surgeons. However, the background and training of surgeons does not permit them to be the "complete" spine practitioner who must unravel the mystery and complexity of the challenge of the lumbar spine. The surgeon's interest and training are built upon surgical technique and structural solutions to a problem that heretofore has belied the purely structural paradigm. The overly simplistic view that structure equals function does not appear to fit the spine model. A countless number of failed spine surgeries, although performed with technical excellence, attests to this fact.

We have also learned that pain is a complex set of events and neuronal interactions that encompasses a combination of excitatory as well as inhibitory influences in the nervous system. Pain is experiential and therefore intrinsically subjective in nature. The search for the cause of pain continues to move away from solely structural explanations toward those implicating biochemical mediators and molecular triggers. The future should bring us a better understanding of the role of inflammation in disc disease. The chemical mediators and molecular triggers that modulate these phenomena should continue to be explored, as they will further add to our understanding of pathogenesis and supply predictive and preventive measures.

Additionally, we must sort out the role of neurotransmitters, such as substance P and VIP, in the pain-relay system. Are these neurotransmitters simply messengers of the pain or are they actual causes of pain? Demonstrating their presence after stimulation of the nociceptive system by a variety of perturbations does nothing more than confirm their role as messengers. However, finding these and other neuropeptides in the annulus of the disc after stimulation of the dorsal root ganglion and the disc demonstrates the central role the intervertebral disc plays in the generation of spinal pain. In addition, research in which the neurons of the dorsal root ganglion and the disc are stimulated offers a vital link to understanding referral pain. Hyperstimulation of receptor neurons with resultant referral zone pain to a site other than the actual site of pain generation can successfully explain the myriad names given to low back syndromes by various practitioners. The multifidus syndrome of the myofascial specialist is the sacroiliac syndrome of the physical therapist, is the subluxation of the chiropractor, is the sacral biomechanical defect of the osteopath, is the back sprain of the general practitioner. Unfortunately this conundrum of nomenclature leads to breakdowns in interdisciplinary communication and confusion relayed to the consumers of health care. This has also led, in my opinion, to some uninterpretable research in spinal disorders, because researchers have lumped all types of pain syndromes into one bold group called "low back pain." This overgeneralization has led to erroneous conclusions and assumptions about low back disorders.

To achieve a successful outcome in the treatment of patients with pain requires a truly holistic approach. Although we must search for the individual pieces of the pain jigsaw puzzle, we must treat each individual as the sum of all the parts.

Why does one patient experience pain apparently from a disc that does not look substantially different from a disc found in a pain-free patient? Do the molecular and biochemical changes that we are now able to identify and measure create the mechanical changes associated with annular disruption and nuclear dehydration, or does mechanical stress lead to the breakdown and secondarily to the liberation of the chemical and neuropeptide molecules? In the future, intradiscal therapy will be molecular in nature and designed to modulate the chemical milieu rather than dissolve, disrupt, or remove portions of the intervertebral disc. Additionally, I predict that there will be means to chemically retard the senescence of intervertebral discs, thereby delaying the onset of the degenerative process and the resultant mechanical changes that secondarily affect the spine. These advances suggest there will be a shifting emphasis in the care of painful spinal disorders toward more responsibility for the nonsurgical practitioner.

As spinal practitioners, we must strive to optimize function instead of solely treating pain. Pain should only be viewed as a deterrent to the patient to attain normal function. Function should therefore be the standard by which all therapeutic interventions should be judged. However, how are we to define function? Is function strength? If so, should this be measured isokinetically or isometrically? Is it enough to test strength of the spinal extensors and rectus abdominis or should the strength of the lower extremities and total body strength be considered as well? Additionally, should we consider lumbar range of motion, muscular endurance, aerobic capacity, physical work capacity, subjective pain rating scales, charts of medication usage, a tabulation of medical dollars spent in post-program aftercare, return-to-work ratios, and recidivism as defined by medical visits and secondary surgery?

Medical decision making is further complicated by requests from employers and insurance companies for objective criteria for functional status. These requests have led to an explosion of high-tech, microprocessor-controlled, data-acquisition systems for testing the muscular strength of the trunk and lumbar range of motion. Unfortunately, even though these systems collect reproducible data, the use of the data remains open to debate and challenge. Agreement upon the definition of function and the criteria by which it should be judged is a mandatory future requirement in spinal care. It is my opinion that function should be defined by a battery of data that are compiled and tabulated on a scorecard. The factors should include the patient's self-rating of function, the patient's self-rating of pain level, work duty status, and annualized expenditures of medical dollars to maintain the functional condition. Additionally, it is my opinion that physiatrists must take the lead in defining functional disability, as they have in other areas such as stroke, head injury, and spinal cord injury. Education of the employers and the insurance companies as to the realistic utility of objective functional assessment is also imperative. Pain remains in its essence an experiential phenomenon and therefore inherently subjective in nature. Therefore, any attempt to concretize this phenomenon is futile unless it takes into consideration the social impact of the pain experience.

Additionally, employers must take a greater responsibility for the burden of the injured worker problem. Poor work conditions, intransigence in modifying work stations, unavailable modified work, inadequate attempts to appropriately match the physical capacity of the employee to the tasks of the job, and occupational dissatisfaction are all issues that are outside the realm and control of the medical establishment. Industry's attempt to save medical dollars by contracting for cut-rate medical care has also led to poor care and secondarily to increased expenditures and employee dissatisfaction, with a concomitant steady increase in litigation-related expenses. Corporate America must be educated that good medical care costs more at the front end, but eventually saves dollars. Additionally, the institution of prevention programs and the modification of work stations and job tasks must be undertaken to successfully combat the issues of the injured worker. The medical establishment must team with corporate America to solve these issues.

Probably the most important advance in the practice of spinal medicine in the last 15 years has been in the arena of imaging. The technology now permits a noninvasive morphologic evaluation of the spine to be undertaken by a nonsurgeon. This is a major step when one considers that before computed tomography the only way to image the spinal contents was through myelography, an imaging technique that made the spine appear as a "black box" that was mysterious and unapproachable. Additionally, the normal myelogram relegated the diagnostician and the patient to the void of "chronic lumbar sprain." What was then even worse was placing the patient into the diagnostic penitentiary designated functional low back pain. This designation is in itself quite interesting, if one considers the context in which "functional" is used—not to connote physical disability and limitation associated with a somatic impairment but rather inferring a psychological state by which the patient created his or her own chronic pain state. Myelography therefore made it very easy for the surgeons to use a very simplistic black or white rating scale of back disorders. Either the patient had an abnormal myelogram and was designated as having a surgical problem, or a normal myelogram and was designated as a nonsurgical spinal disorder that in the surgeon's mind required no definitive treatment (i.e., "It's now someone else's problem. Having surgery can't help").

With the advent of modern imaging techniques, coupled with the marvelous advances in selective injections guided by digital fluoroscopy, the ball game has changed. Now subtleties can be analyzed, and provocatory procedures to piece together the pain jigsaw puzzle have become powerful and necessary tools of the diagnostician. Additionally, the role of the spinal diagnostician has emerged. This individual is not necessarily a surgeon, and I believe it is best not to be the surgical team member. This new species of practitioner is a mixture of radiologist, physiatrist, anesthesiologist, internist, and psychobehaviorist. It is my belief and contention that the well-trained physiatrist should be able to be the central player and team leader of this diagnostic powerhouse.

Spinal imaging should be undertaken under the direction of a radiologist with subspecialty interest in the spine. The general radiologist who interprets the occasional scan cannot help to the same degree the subspecialty spinal radiologist can. Additionally, the radiologist must become part of the diagnostic team. He or she must become a true consultant and not a blind reader of scans who only supplies neatly transcribed copies of their interpretations. By involving the radiologist, the clinician can enrich his or her understanding of morphology while the radiologist learns how to analyze problems as a clinician. It is imperative for the radiologist to learn to interpret imaging studies without a "surgical" bias. Reports that contain the words "surgical disc lesion," or "clinically insignificant stenosis" do not belong on any report. Radiologists are morphologists, and only the clinician can place the structural findings into perspective. Therefore the notion of false positive imaging studies is a misconception. Morphologic findings may be found to be asymptomatic, but they are present and can therefore not be designated as "false positives." What is there is there. It is the clinician's responsibility to properly analyze all of the diagnostic data and carefully construct the clinical picture by placing all of the pieces of the diagnostic jigsaw puzzle into their proper locations.

The correlative use of diagnostic blocks will be further expanded in the future. There will be increasing demand for more precise information to classify diagnoses into more refined categories. The surgeries that are planned will require this precision of diagnosis to achieve success.

Traditional spine practitioners have begun to explore the avenues of manual therapy. Manual medicine most certainly has a place in the armamentarium of spinal practice. However, the timing of its application and the amount of emphasis it deserves in the overall treatment plan have not been clearly defined. The trend in treatment of spinal disorders continues to move towards active participatory patient care rather than passive means. Patients are becoming more aware of treatment options and are therefore becoming better consumers of health care. The physician's duty must encompass a strong component of patient education. Similar to the educational effort that accompanies rehabilitation of the spinal cord injured patient, the spinal pain patient requires extensive educational programming. The patient's pain is heightened by fear of catastrophic disability. Unfortunately the seed for this destructive thought process was most often planted by comments such as, "If you don't have something done right away, you'll have permanent nerve damage," or "You have degenerative disc disease and nothing can be done to treat this condition." These types of comments spoken to patients are thoughtless and inherently destructive by the very nature of what they connote.

Chiropractors and physiatrists must learn to develop a better working relationship. Patients must be given more options than (1) improving with chiropractic care or (2) facing surgery, such as is often the case in many communities. With better teaming, patients can have the opportunity to be exposed to the entire gamut of available nonoperative treatments before considering the possibility of surgery.

Additionally, the working relationship between physical therapists and physicians must improve. This will require physicians to become more involved in the rehabilitation of their patients. To send the patient to the physical therapist with a prescription that reads "evaluate and treat" is inappropriate in my opinion. The physician must supply a diagnosis that will often continue to evolve in its specificity over the course of the treatment plan. As the diagnosis becomes more refined, so does the treatment plan. The therapist must communicate to the physician when the patient is not progressing and not wait 6 weeks for the next follow-up visit. Early communication can speed recovery and reduce medical expenditures by allowing constructive changes to occur in the treatment algorithm. For instance the patient with radicular pain secondary to a herniated intervertebral disc might benefit from an epidural cortisone injection rather than have 3 more weeks of traction, manipulation, massage, and other modalities. This intervention can, for example, shorten the pain-control phase of treatment and allow for the early institution of an active training and education program.

Another area where the future will need to bring further clarification is in the area of acceleration-deceleration cervical injuries. "Whiplash" injuries remain one of the more difficult clinical problems the physician faces. Not only are we called upon to diagnose the condition, but we are asked to clearly define causation. This, unfortunately, is a role that many find uncomfortable. Additionally, we often find ourselves forced into asking questions as an investigative detective rather than a treating physician. Our role is not to gather information for the attorneys but rather to treat our patients effectively. Considerable debate remains within the scientific establishment regarding the structural and pathologic consequences of acceleration-deceleration injuries. The type, timing, and quantity of treatment prescribed varies from practitioner to practitioner and even from country to country. An increased understanding of annular disc injuries that occur secondary to this injury mechanism certainly sheds light upon the reason why so many patients remain symptomatic for great lengths of time following vehicular trauma. It also can explain the delayed onset of intervertebral disc herniation with the development of radiculopathy that may occur 3–6 months following an accident. This phenomenon probably represents a gradual disc prolapse syndrome, in which the injured annular fibers gradually attenuate and tear, leading to nuclear migration and resultant nerve root inflammation. The pain may therefore evolve from a dorsal primary ramus syndrome of axial pain and vague, fleeting referral zone discomfort into the proximal portion of the extremity to true radicular pain into the extremity, often accompanied by a lessening of the neck pain itself. Defining causation, therefore, will require a better understanding of spinal pathoanatomy and pathophysiology.

The future of spinal medicine does appear bright and exciting. However, it will require the dedication of able and bright physicians to the study of painful spinal disorders. Additionally, it will require the teaming of appropriately trained physiatrists, surgeons, radiologists, psychiatrists, anesthesiologists, internists, physical therapists, and chiropractors in a multidisciplinary effort directed toward solving this complex spectrum of problems.

INDEX

Entries in **boldface type** indicate complete chapters.